PHYSICAL
DISOBEDIENCE

PHYSICAL DISOBEDIENCE

AN UNRULY GUIDE TO
HEALTH &
STAMINA
FOR THE
MODERN
FEMINIST

SARAH HAYS COOMER

SEAL PRESS

Seal Press

Hachette Book Group

1290 Avenue of the Americas, New York, NY 10104

SealPress.com

@sealpress

Printed in the United States of America

First Edition: August 2018

Published by Seal Press, an imprint of Perseus Books, LLC, a subsidiary of Hachette Book Group, Inc. The Seal Press name and logo is a trademark of the Hachette Book Group.

The publisher is not responsible for websites (or their content) that are not owned by the publisher.

Valarie Kaur speech quote on page 41 is Copyright © 2016 by Valarie Kaur.

Jason Isbell lyrics used with permission

Dead Horses lyrics used with permission

Quote from *Griefwalker*, a documentary film of Tim Wilson produced by the National Film Board of Canada © 2008

Print book interior design by Amy Quinn.

Library of Congress Cataloging-in-Publication Data has been applied for.

ISBNs: 978-1-58005-773-8 (paperback), 978-1-58005-774-5 (ebook)

LSC-C

10 9 8 7 6 5 4 3 2 1

For everyone who has ever felt like a puffer fish

Contents

Author's Note

The names and identifying details of people mentioned by first name only in this book have been changed to protect the innocent. Body baggage can be a dirty business, but the stories that follow—the ones these anonymous souls were graciously willing to share—have steadied me and readied me to be a crime-fighting, bullshit-bashing, comfy-cozy-wearing ninja. Named or unnamed, they will do the same for you.

"Disobedience is the true foundation of liberty."

—Henry David Thoreau,
Civil Disobedience

PART 1

BEAUTY UNHINGED

CHAPTER 1

Strange Beauty

It's picture time, ladies! Smile pretty! Suck it in. Keep it tight. Arms on hips. Twist your body. Bend those knees. You know how we do. If you're small enough and easy enough on the eyes and ears, you'll blend right in.

• • •

Nope. Not anymore. We're in the middle of a heavy lift here, and we're going to need our legs under us.

There is precisely zero chance we will be able to achieve equal stature while chronically apologizing for our own perfectly healthy, unconventionally beautiful bodies.

Women have made enormous progress over the last two hundred years for gender equality and human rights. The feminist activists who came before us deserve ticker tape parades and a series of provocative documentary films in their honor. Sojourner Truth, Betty Friedan, Gloria Steinem, Shirley Chisholm, Diane Nash, and countless others were unrepentant revolutionaries, doing the dirtiest work long before our time. They were bold and relentless—and they deserve better than what we are doing to our bodies today. They deserve us at our strongest. We've come a long way, but after all this time, we remain enshrined in hourglass, whisper-thin ideals perpetuated not only by the media but by our own acquiescence.

We have a mountain of work yet to do on a whole range of issues. You know the ones: equal pay, affordable health care, stronger gun laws, paid family leave, equal representation in government and business, criminal justice, financial reform, support for immigrant and refugee families, environmental conservation, preventing violence against women, minorities, and the disabled, and on and on. It's a hell of a list.

We understand the work that needs to be done to advance human rights on a macro level. Movements are taking shape worldwide. Women of every ethnicity are running for office and standing up for disenfranchised people in all walks of life, but if we aren't grounded in our bodies in the first place, none of it will stick. As foot soldiers, we must do the work, on a micro level, to shift the conversations in our own minds and to feed our bodies.

Women are, and will continue to be, at the heart of progressive change throughout the world. We vote in greater numbers than men. We invest tirelessly in our own educations and those of our kids, and we advocate for public health and safety policies that benefit the community as a whole. But before we can make seismic professional, economic, and sociological changes, we have to squeeze out of our Spanx and remember how it feels to breathe—with sweat in our eyes, air in our lungs, and music pouring boldly from our speakers.

This book is a manual for how to bring our activism home, into our bodies, by way of pleasurable, purposeful self-care.

Physical Disobedience is any action that feeds, strengthens, or nurtures our bodies as a direct, unapologetic act of defiance. It is fierce appreciation for what our bodies can do, how they feel, and how they look in all of their "imperfect" glory. It's a concrete, immediately impactful way to push back that benefits each of us as individuals while simultaneously effecting positive, social change. In other words, taking care of our bodies is a form of political action.

Physical Disobedience is about refusing to acquiesce, refusing to allow our bodies to be objectified by others, and taking a hard look at how we objectify them ourselves. It is feminism via fitness. We know how to care for the people we love. We need to make sure our own bodies are cared for as well, and that requires a hefty dose of appreciation and exploration. There is too much at stake. Our bodies make our work possible. Reducing them to decorative trinkets reduces our impact and destroys our experience of being alive.

• • •

What do beauty, health, and power look like? According to popular memes, they look like pouty lips and bony shoulders. These images are well defined for us. They are the driving force behind the contorted rituals we inflict on ourselves in the name of glamour, but chronic dieting and unrelenting feelings of failure are the furthest thing from beautiful. They are ugly and damaging, and they sap us of vital energy.

The notions imbedded in our minds about our bodies not measuring up, and all the menial tasks we must undertake to make them submit, eat away at our ability to do what needs to be done.

If we want to move on to the next phase of humanity where women have *at least* a 50 percent share in governance from the school board to the presidency—because *duh*—we need to surgically remove these notions, one at a time, learning as we go to hear the physical messages being transmitted through our body systems—of pain, anxiety, fear, and fatigue—and address them head on with endorphins and fresh air, rather than burying them in fad diets or cinnamon crumb cake.

MAKING PEACE

The summer after I graduated from college I spent sunny afternoons in a dark, one-room apartment, staring at my body in a plastic, full-length mirror that was stuck to my closet door with double-sided tape.

The bottom left corner was always detaching from the door. I nudged it with my toe, and it would stick for a moment before—pop—coming loose again.

When I engaged in this charming self-analysis, I was usually wearing some incarnation of faded polyester lace underwear and no bra. I faced the mirror head on, eyes narrow, stance wide, and let my breath go, watching flesh spill out over the elastic edges of my panties.

I took stock. *Boobs sagging. Belly rolls. Disgusting thighs. I can't believe I'm wasting my life in this body.*

I picked up my camera and snapped photos, front and side. I wished someone were there to take a picture of my cellu-butt, but no such luck. *Probably for the best. Nobody wants to see that anyway.*

I printed the pictures out and posted them on the refrigerator door. *Gross.* I figured if I could see for myself how revolting I was, I would find the motivation to do something about it.

I was twenty-two years old, five foot seven inches, 155 pounds. Seriously.

That boring, overworked pattern went on for years. I took on diets and "challenges" to get my appetite and "body fat" under control. I planned workouts that sometimes happened, sometimes not, and cooked a bunch of vegetables that generally ended up in the trash a week later, slimy in Tupperware.

I hovered a hair-trigger above a state of panic, like SpongeBob SquarePants having a nervous breakdown at the sight of cake or fries or food of any kind.

Even when I lost weight, the result never seemed beautiful. It never fit the image I had in my head of how I was supposed to look, how a powerful, confident woman should look—thin, graceful, cheekbones for days, narrow limbs, and a liquid stare.

That woman haunted me, a ghostly image I cobbled together from the usual suspects: billboards, movies, and fashion magazines. She hovered in my mind in every clothing store and at every buffet

I attended from the age of fifteen to thirty-five, reminding me in no uncertain terms that I did not measure up. Her giant eyes, baggy sweaters, and skinny jeans beckoned: "You can be beautiful if you just control yourself. Deprive yourself a little more. Find the right boots and lipstick, the right super-cute workout gear, and you will have arrived. You're a wreck. Lose the weight."

It was whiplash, predictable and pointless: weight loss and gain, cleanses, makeovers, diets, and half-hearted attempts at trending fashions. The obsession with manipulating my body in one way or another monopolized my bank account, my free time, and my brain year after famished year.

My body was fine. It was more than fine. It was young and strong, but I spent two decades weakening it while shortchanging every other aspect of my life. The fight took me to my knees in front of toilets. It plagued me with stomach ulcers and depression. It prevented me from speaking my mind in social situations and asserting myself in professional ones, and it stopped me from exploring pleasures and possibilities that would otherwise have been open to me.

I've tried to guess how many hours a day, in the thick of those years, I spent feeling awkward in my clothes and obsessing about food or exercise, but truthfully, I don't think there was any time at all when my body and its inadequacies weren't at least a little bit on my mind.

I've tried to calculate what difference it might have made in my career, relationships, income, and mental and physical health if those years had been spent differently.

But there is no going back to those summer afternoons in my discount underwear. I can't recapture the time that was lost. I can't reach out to lovers I drove away by putting down my body and looking to them for reassurance. I can't retrieve mislaid job opportunities and vanished friendships.

It has been eighteen years since that summer in front of the mirror, and I'm relieved to have spent much of that time peeling off sheets of soot and ash covering my eyes—one brittle, filmy layer at a time.

I didn't become a personal trainer to lose weight or to get ultra fit. I have never been to a 6 a.m. boot camp, and I have never run more than a 5K. I still eat all the treats my temperamental stomach will allow in reasonable portions. I'm able to steer clear of the guilt-driven binges that used to torment me because I know that tomorrow and the day after that I'll have the chance to enjoy food again. There is no need to stuff myself when I'm not playing a daily game of deprivation and negotiation.

I became a personal trainer because I wanted to extend an olive branch to my body, to find a way to live with it, and through it, gratefully. I couldn't bear the thought of an entire lifetime spent hating the physical vehicle that I could not, under any circumstances, escape. So I set out to mend my body (and my opinion of it) and became a trainer for people like me, people who want to make peace with their bodies and get stronger and more powerful along the way.

Working with my personal training clients has taught me what beauty actually looks like, and it's not at all what I thought. It is strange and mysterious. It is honest, well-worn, and radiant.

I had no idea how far removed I was from true beauty and feminine power until I could begin to see them for what they are, but I can tell you now, with eyes *almost* clear, that it's mighty fine on the other side of that illusion.

A journalist asked me once how I justify being a personal trainer when I talk so much about treating bodies of all sizes as intuitive, bright resources for leadership and connection. She thought that because I'm a trainer, my job is to help people mold their bodies "into shape." In a way, she was right. I do help people mold their bodies, but not into any particular shape. I'm not trying to make them fit any picture that has ever been printed anywhere. I'm helping them discover what their bodies feel like when they are able to stand up, know their own worth, and stop diminishing what they have to offer. And that can come at any weight.

RECOGNIZING BEAUTY

Leonard Cohen wrote, "When you call me close to tell me your body is not beautiful, I want to summon the eyes and hidden mouths of stone and light and water to testify against you."[1]

When I see capable, intelligent human beings belittling themselves based on looking not fill-in-the-blank enough, I want to testify. Actually, I want to scream. Assuming they're not cruel, self-involved people, the only ugly thing about them is their unceasing tendency to undervalue their bodies and contributions.

Every time you knock yourself down a notch because your hair isn't straight enough or your backside isn't small enough, you are laying waste to mental energy that could be spent doing something useful or enjoyable—or doing nothing at all but listening to the birds chirp and watching clouds float by. A lifetime spent merely *enduring* your body squanders your power and forfeits your capacity for contentment. But a lifetime spent living into and through your body frees you to be a whole person, with valid needs and concerns, regardless of the size you wear or the uniqueness of your individual style.

When my clients deride themselves for not measuring up to the images in their own minds, when they shrink from personal and professional growth because they believe their bodies disqualify them from advancement, I ache, again, to testify to the extraordinary strength I see in them. They are intelligent and wise and ridiculous, and I adore them.

When I ask them about the women they love—about their mothers, sisters, partners, and best friends—they testify. They tell me about perseverance, intelligence, and humor. But when dealing with their own bodies, the grace they offer their loved ones dissolves in a swamp of irrelevant criteria that they apply to no one but themselves.

Beauty has nothing to do with the pursuit of "perfection." Beauty is found in authenticity, empathy, play, and passion. It is found in our humanity—bodies at work, limber and awake, free and unbowed.

But most of us can't see any of that. All we can see are the numbers on the scale, the pictures on the fridge, the dieting apps on our phones, and the plastic mirrors taped to the door—pop—day after day, year after year.

We're trying to look like something that has nothing to do with who we are, and that's not beautiful. It's a prison sentence for every woman who has ever been disregarded, underpaid, assaulted, or ignored.

Nip and tuck, ladies, or lose your place in line.

We have been looking for validation in the wrong places all along, and that backward search has cost us dearly, stripping us of opportunities, cold hard cash, and well-deserved confidence. Worst of all, it has led us to exploit, control, and shun our bodies—which makes us sick, body and mind. And feeling sick keeps us quiet. It keeps us distracted and dependent on somebody else for approval. It keeps us grumpy when we should be having the time of our lives while our bodies are younger than they will ever be again.

The reasons we have pursued diet and exercise have been misguided at best and destructive at worst. The big, illusive promise of achieving some kind of skin-and-bones victory over ourselves is a lie. I've lost the weight, and I've seen a lot of other people lose it, too. That alone doesn't do the trick. Skinny doesn't make for happy, folks.

When we find new, powerful, healthy ways to be in our bodies—large or small—we are beautiful and free, but when we throw everything we have into defeating our bodies, we find nothing but an empty void at the bottom of a bone-dry well. And we wake up skinny and parched. Or, more likely, fat and parched.

Being thin doesn't legitimize us. Caring about something and doing something about it does. Celebrating and commiserating with friends and lovers does. Using whatever energy we can muster to make a difference for somebody who needs a boost—that's where legitimacy comes from.

• • •

So what *does* beauty look like?

It looks like Lisa, who spends her days as a social worker in underfunded public schools. Lisa goes to work every day under an avalanche of bureaucracy. Many of her students suffer on the streets or in abusive homes. She comforts them the best she can and goes home at night to two kids of her own. She ruminates on what more she can do to give her students a little bit more of a shot, to expose and heal the bigotry they face on a daily basis. She spends her weekends sponsoring birthday parties for foster kids who want to be an astronaut or a princess for the day and throwing baby showers for teenage moms she mentors. During football season, she eats brisket and tacos every chance she gets while cheering on her beloved Longhorns.

Lisa is beauty.

It looks like Janine, who runs operations for a major entertainment company in Hollywood, California, while raising a daughter and stepson. She is a former hellion who somehow found herself president of her daughter's elementary school PTA. She has opened her arms to a family of three generations living next door in a two-bedroom house. She lets the whole neighborhood full of kids and grandkids run roughshod through her home every day, feeding them and giving them a safe place to crash when pressurized family dynamics explode. She is a fierce defender of women's and LGBTQ rights, a hiker, and a one-woman wrecking ball against the anti-vaccine movement.

Janine is beauty.

It looks like Amber, a forty-five-year-old physician who has worked her entire career to achieve a place of professional respect that allows her to choose which committees to chair, which research projects to pursue, and which causes to support. When a colleague ignored her repeated insistence that she was not interested in doing his work for him (and giving him the credit), she wrote a scathing letter to him and his superior outlining exactly what her interests were; how she planned to spend her time in the coming months; and when she would be unavailable on vacation. They acquiesced. She had done the work.

She knew her value. She recognized when she was being disrespected, and she called bullshit.

Amber is beauty.

And it looks like Janay Jumping Eagle, a Native American student at Little Wound High School on the Pine Ridge Reservation near the Badlands of South Dakota. Her Lakota tribe suffered from a rash of teen suicides in recent years, and she took matters into her own hands, by reaching out to kids who were coming up in grades behind her with an event called There Is Hope. The event featured a basketball tournament, food for the kids (many of whom can't afford a full meal every day), suicide prevention booths, and first-person storytelling from parents who lost their children.

Janay said, "After losing so many friends and family members, I just wanted to make a positive impact on my community. I wanted other people to know that there are people who care and who will help with whatever they need. I was just thinking what can I do? What do these kids like to do the most? And I thought of basketball. I knew the kids were safe and happy playing basketball. They were smiling at the end of the day, and that's all I wanted. The suicide rate dropped after that, so I think it worked. I like that I was a part of that. I just wanted to help."

She appeared in a 2017 documentary called *Little Wounds' Warriors*.[2] She is just a seventeen-year-old kid, growing up in a tribe steeped in poverty, alcoholism, and cultural injustice, but she understands viscerally that healing can come from moving our bodies and connecting with our communities.

Janay is beauty.

· · ·

Whatever the shape of our flesh, the color of our skin, or the "imperfections" we perceive in ourselves, there is nothing that matters more than being as connected and present as we can and as astonished as we can to be alive and well. The more we live into our passions, the more we settle into our bodies and the more our bodies begin to serve our purposes.

Physical Disobedience is about defiance, but it is not about anger. Above all else, it's a celebration of rowdy women and an exploration of how to harness our physical and emotional prowess for good. It's a salute to smarts, goofiness, softness, and muscle.

There is power in unconventional beauty and even more power in recognizing it.

Our bodies need not comply. They belong to us. They are the greatest tools we have to enhance and reinforce every aspect of our lives, and it is long past time to write our own definitions of beauty, for ourselves.

RESPONDING TO OUTRAGE

"Mom! Run!" My son shouted, "We have to go around three times without falling!" We were standing on a concrete track that borders a field behind a school near our house. We took off and made it three-quarters of the way around before he declared breathlessly, "And we can walk whenever we need to, Ma."

I hadn't run in months. I don't like running, never have, but for my little guy on the first spring afternoon of the year, for that moment, I would do anything. So we ran. We paused to walk for a minute before he took off again, leaving me with my thoughts, *I can't believe they want to slash funding for the Addiction and Recovery Act (CARA)*[3]. *I mean who the hell doesn't want addicts in every town in America getting off opioids?!* Despair washed over me—bleak and abrasive—but my son caught my eye up ahead with an impish smile, and I was off again.

Chest out, running uphill in flatfooted Converse, it dawned on me. This is it. This is the plan. When the horror show of partisanship, racism, misogyny, and class warfare descends, my reaction, every time, needs to be to run up hills, a few thousand feet until I can breathe and see the sky again; or drop for a set of impromptu park bench push-ups; or whip up a few servings of curried cauliflower with almonds and golden raisins, for the first time ever.

The balms that will heal our bodies and minds—and give us the strength to shovel the truckloads of short-sighted, asinine, toxic waste arriving daily at our doorsteps—are oxygen and vital nutrients, the building blocks of our human bodies.

Each step and every healthy bite takes us closer to well-being, closer to raw, unrepentant liberty at home, at work, in our neighborhoods, and within the confines of our own minds.

When you can't breathe for the state of the news and your muscles ache from grief pulsing just below the surface of your skin, defy the urge to placate yourself with sugar and screens. Lash out against the people and policies causing you pain by activating your body and claiming your physical space. It doesn't matter if you are wheelchair bound or muscle bound. Whatever the state of your body, begin each day with naked appreciation for your unkempt hair, your biceps, quadriceps, and the intercostal muscles that enable your ribs to breathe in and out. Make time to move for the sake of personal liberty. Dress in clothes that feel dynamic and easy, and practice sitting, walking, and standing in ways that feel expansive—deviant even. Disobey the rules you've embraced that dictate how you carry yourself through the world, and uproot your habitual responses to adversity.

With political and personal fires cropping up all over the horizon, your job is to make sure you're hydrated, well-rested, equipped with protective gear, and ready with a pick ax to build an impenetrable fireline—knowing all along that you've never been more beautiful or more powerful. This book will help you suit up.

We have to stop apologizing for our bodies, and we will only be able to do that when we associate beauty with purpose. Effortlessly.

True beauty is ours for the taking. To begin reclaiming it, we must be able to stand up, tall and grounded—and for that, we will need the muscles at our core. We will need our hearts and lungs to process air as efficiently as possible; legs ready to catapult us forward;

and arms robust enough to lift whatever needs lifting. We will need our strength in whatever capacity each of us can manage. And we will need each other—including and especially the compelling, brave, wholehearted, and provocative men who have our backs.

There is power in our bodies and in our numbers.

And the best part is, we can walk whenever we need to.

◇◇

Fill in the Fact

The thing I hate most about my body is _____

_____.

I have felt this way since _____

_____.

Fixating on this "problem" has made my life (circle one):
Better   Worse

If I didn't think about how ugly this body part is for an entire week, I would have more time and brainpower for _____

_____.

Beauty is _____

_____.

My friend _____ is beautiful because _____

_____.

◇◇

There is precisely zero chance we
will be able to achieve equal stature
while chronically apologizing
for our own perfectly healthy,
unconventionally beautiful bodies.

CHAPTER 2

Holding On to Air

Standing on the sidewalk on a sunny, early-summer afternoon, the kid from next door came tumbling over to me, all long limbs and panting breath. "Did you know you can't hold on to air??" she asked.

"I did know that!" I replied, "you try and grab it, but, *DAHH!*, it slips away." We tried and failed and tried even harder, but no—we couldn't hold on to air. Sorely disappointed though we were, we shrugged it off and parted ways until next time.

In the days following that astute observation from mini-Yoda next door, I began to catch myself—with alarming regularity—holding on to air, attempting to control the uncontrollable. I grasped and grabbed and lurched in an impossible effort to "get a handle" on various situations. But trying to hold on to air is like trying to hold on to summer or, of course, beauty. It can't be done. As soon as you try to grab it or re-create it, it slips beyond your grasp.

This holds true for everything we cherish: love, success, freedom, money, or time. The tighter we hold on, the more we find ourselves trapped by paranoia at the thought of losing it—and, in that trap, we lose access to the very comfort we craved in the first place. It slips away like air through our fingers.

The world we live in demands that we take "control" of our circumstances, including and especially our bodies, but when we compare our spectacularly human bodies to manufactured, ephemeral, photoshopped images, we set ourselves up to fail mightily in comparison. This "failure" takes a heavy toll on our confidence and that, in turn, impacts every other aspect of our lives: personal, professional, or otherwise. When we try to emulate fabricated images, we are quite literally holding on to air. And when we punish ourselves for not achieving those impossible aims, we weaken ourselves—and delegitimize our value as intelligent beings beyond our physical appearances.

We can't pixelate our bodies. We can't reshape real-life saddlebags with the wave of a cursor any more than we can stop time by closing our eyes, covering our ears, and singing *LALALALA* at the top of our lungs.

So—as we discussed in the last chapter—if beauty isn't what we thought it was, if, instead, it is an amorphous concept that has more to do with achieving vitality and reinforcing our power than producing sucked-in, draped-over, painted-on replicas of our better selves, how can we divorce ourselves from the toxic belief systems and behavior patterns that have held so many of us prisoner for most of our lives?

The first step is to recognize that manipulation of our bodies in service of mythical, standardized ideals is an illness. It's a destructive infatuation that dilutes our influence.

WASTING AWAY

When I was just a few years older than my neighbor friend, barely out of high school, I spent the money I had saved continuously from eighteen birthdays and Christmases to go to Europe with a volunteer organization that offered short-term assignments around the world.

I signed up to work half the summer at an orphanage in Poland and the other half at a refugee camp in Switzerland. I loved the idea of traveling as a volunteer and wanted to break out of my isolated, teenage bubble. I understood in an oblique way that my vision of the world was limited and wanted to see what I was missing.

The reasons for my trip seemed selfless from a distance. I wanted to help some kids. That much was true, but the deeper truth was that the whole adventure was constructed around a selfish motive: to allow for a pilgrimage. I wanted to travel, yes, but specifically, I wanted to go to Auschwitz, the concentration camp.

There was no logical explanation for this. I have no Jewish blood. My family didn't know anyone who died there. I had many Jewish friends growing up, but none of them were getting on a plane bound for Poland.

Still, I was drawn to it—the darkness of the place, the wasting away of vibrant bodies, and the destruction of life for no reason other than blind hatred. Obsessed with shrinking my own body or otherwise disguising it, I knew my fixation was unhealthy but couldn't shake it. I was desperately trying to hold on to air, to a portrait of beauty not reflected by my unwieldy, postadolescent body. I wish there was a better word than *body* for the beast I was inhabiting at the time because, to me, it was a vessel, a prison cell of repugnant flesh.

I wanted to be in a place where everyone could agree that food is vital and deprivation is sick, so I went to find out what neglected bodies look like. I wanted a reason to value my body instead of despising it. I needed to find out why I should not strive to be like those emaciated people in the photos. I was ashamed to be so fascinated with Auschwitz but needed to see for myself that wasting bodies are not beautiful; they are an ugly waste of human potential.

I went looking in the darkness for the light.

I could write forever about the atrocities that took place at Auschwitz and the memorials erected there, but I will spare you the graphic details. You know most of them already. The horrors extended well beyond the gas chambers to starvation and suffocation cells, firing squads, and crematoria. The photographic evidence is haunting, and the rooms full of shoes, glasses, and human hair that were left behind are unsettling reminders of the valuable and very real lives that were extinguished.

At the entrance stands that famous gate with the words atop it "ARBEIT MACHT FREI," *Work will set you free*, but, of course, weakened bodies, stripped of nutrients and self-determination can't accomplish much at all. People weren't brought there to work; they were brought there to disappear.

Sick as I was, disappearing seemed preferable to being chubby.

As I left Auschwitz, just outside the exit, there was a small refreshment stand selling sausages and potato chips. My stomach turned—not because they were selling food in such a place or because I had subsisted for the past two days on Snickers bars and orange soda that tasted like lollipops—I was sick because after all I'd seen that day, when I walked outside and saw that refreshment stand, I still hated myself for wanting that food.

People suffered and died there. I came to learn from their pain but walked out with the same twisted ping-pong game playing in my head. The appetites that rose up from my body were to be extinguished at all costs; I had no ability to distinguish craving from hunger; and my jean shorts still fit all wrong.

A few miles down the road at Birkenau, also known as Auschwitz II, train tracks stretch from the outside world, through the center of a long narrow building, and into the heart of a vast, open space, surrounded by barbed wire fencing and speckled with gray, squat buildings—some still standing and some reduced to rubble by fire and time. When the Nazis left the camp behind, they burned what they could and abandoned the rest. The Polish government left the camp just as they found it.

The day was beautiful, sunny, and warm, a stark, yawning landscape. It felt like an Oklahoma skyline—flat, open, and bathed in light.

I wandered around, peering out over the camp from the watchtower and exploring the bunks where adults and children carved their prayers and rememberances. I stood at the edge of the pond where they threw the ashes of the dead as trees stretched peacefully overhead and leaves rustled in a gentle, steady breeze.

My attempt at shock therapy had failed. I wasn't okay with my body yet, far from it. I still pined to be skin and bones. I spent the rest of the summer teaching music and art classes to kids who had seen more war, loneliness, and disease in their short lives than I will probably ever see in mine. Through it all, I hid Nutella in my suitcase, binged on pasta when I could find it, and shredded photos of myself for having what I perceived as "fatty knees." By obsessing about my own body, I lost the opportunity in front of me to focus on the kids and explore a new place with fresh eyes.

The trip wasn't a total loss. The kids had fun for a few weeks, and, without a doubt, I was changed by the people I met and the circumstances they faced. But how much more could I have learned and contributed if I wasn't busy hiding food from fellow volunteers and worrying about how my legs were positioned on the floor, on the futon, and under the kitchen table?

The potential we squander by picking our bodies to pieces is catastrophic.

The intellectual and psychological resources wasted during my teenage wanderings were miniscule in comparison with the millions of ways we, as women, shortchange ourselves based on whatever we perceive to be wrong with our bodies. It is reflected in our incomes, our intimate relationships, the laws and politicians that govern us, and our ability to advocate for our own rights and the rights of populations in need all over the world. vWhen we hesitate to jump or run on the beach for fear of quivering cellulite, we miss out on Frisbee. We miss out on boogie boarding. We miss out on sand sculptures of hatchling sea turtles headed for the ocean, lovingly crafted by old hippies just a little farther up the beach. And when we stand in a conference room or at a cocktail party with arms folded protectively over our midsections, we disinvite open conversation with peers and potential colleagues; we lose opportunities to connect, innovate, and organize.

We have been bamboozled into believing that our bodies are unacceptable. Beauty has been defined for us, and we have swallowed that definition whole. We are choking on it. It has cut off our airways and gagged us. We need to perform the Heimlich, fling ourselves over the nearest stiff-backed chair, grab each other by the rib cage, and tug with all our might.

Learning to appreciate the function and dignity of our bodies is a discipline.

We have a choice in the way we perceive and care for our bodies, and we can't demand respect from others until we offer it up to ourselves. We can't blame the media for what they're serving up if we continue to buy in. We can't blame the opposite sex for holding our bodies to impossible standards if we are doing the same to ourselves. We do not have to continue grasping at thin air. We can choose different idols.

We human beings have a tendency to compare ourselves to others, to how we used to be or how we would like to be. It's a natural impulse that has been grossly distorted by the prevalence of social media. But since smartphones are here to stay, instead of trying to shut that impulse down, we can use it for good. We can shift our focus away from our own bodies, onto the bodies of women all around us who are getting things done—women we love and admire who are using their bodies, of all sizes, to accomplish ordinary and spectacular achievements in every field imaginable. We may not always be able to make sense of our own bodies, but we can see clearly when it comes to theirs. And that's a worthy place to start.

To defy the absurd, cookie-cutter ideals that have been set out for us—and that we have willingly adopted as our own—we need to stop looking down at ourselves and look *out* at the people around us who exhibit strength, compassion, and leadership. Do we care that Queen Latifah isn't a size 4? Do we care if Brene Brown puts on a few pounds? Do we snipe that Caroline Kennedy needs to eat more? No. We witness and honor them for the examples they set.

Think about the women who inspire you. What do you see when

you look at Maya Angelou, Elizabeth Warren, Kamala Harris, Melissa McCarthy, Mindy Kaling, Adele, or Laila Ali? I'm guessing you don't love your greatest teachers and mentors any less because of the shape of their waists or thighs.

Many of the women we admire have drunk the bad body image Kool-Aid as well, disparaging their bodies in private before gathering up their public faces and heading out to conquer the world. But it's easy for us, from a distance, to see the magnificent, essential people that they are. It's easy for us to lift them up, and the more we focus on respecting their bodies, just as they are, the easier it becomes to respect our own—daily, authentically, and without a second thought.

• • •

My trip to Poland was the beginning of a lifelong practice of appreciating and honoring human bodies for being what they are and doing what they can do. The result of that practice over the past twenty years—to recognize the gorgeous utility of functional and disabled bodies alike—has completely transformed my relationship with my own. It has transformed the way I perceive myself visually and the ways I treat my body—with care, with support, and with a solid dose of gratitude and guts.

Our physical capabilities are incredible expressions of nature at its best, at its sharpest and most practical. Our bodies will serve our ambitions if we feed them with real food and regular movement, instead of stripping them of nutrients and depriving them of the opportunity to get stronger because we are so panicked about how they look.

There is nothing beautiful or healthy about forcing our bodies to submit.

The whole pursuit is madness. It's a cesspool of lost potential, as futile as holding on to air. We are grasping for something that isn't real and doesn't matter. By doing so, we cut our professional and personal objectives off at the knees.

Give your body the tools it needs to be strong, not small. Set it free to be whatever it is at its most lively and unruly. Stand up straight: chest out, body proud. You have rich, long, powerful muscles that wrap up, down, and all the way around your abdomen. This is the core I mentioned at the end of the last chapter. It is the source of your strength, along with powerful arms and legs to carry you through the world and elevate those who need a lift.

We, as women, are the furthest thing from helpless, and writing our bodies off as repugnant because we carry more weight than a supermodel depletes us of all of our authority.

NATURAL RESOURCES

The most overt tests of female strength are, of course, pregnancy and childbirth. And having a baby is one moment in life when we lose all control, when all of the illusions we have about managing our bodies and the circumstances around us fall away. Our bodies take over, and we are abruptly, utterly incapable of holding on to air.

Whatever your personal feelings are about having kids, we can all recognize that giving birth is an incredible feat of endurance and strength. Some will tell you it is magical—not so much for me, though I have done it once myself. It's certainly transformative. There's no doubt about that, but you won't find me tiptoeing through the tulips in my mind when I think of going into labor. Having a child is by no means a necessary rite of passage for womanhood, but we can learn essential lessons by recognizing this visceral and exclusively female experience.

Childbearing isn't my favorite topic (more on that crippling fear in Chapter 9), but having coached many women through their pregnancies, I do see childbirth as a challenging experience that can show us two very important things:

1. What our bodies are capable of if we get out of the way
2. Subversive, unexpected sources of female power

To shed light on this, I spoke with Ami Burnham, a midwife who has been working in her field for over a decade. I wanted to see if I could identify the ways women move through the experience of giving birth and what qualities make for the least traumatic, most treasured birth experiences.

Ami believes that the two greatest disciplines we can take from childbirth are patience and surrender. "I learned about patience and surrender from years of watching so many women and families go through this process," she says. "The patience piece is obvious because you don't have control over when labor starts, how it proceeds, or when it's going to end. You have to be patient with your body, the baby, and the whole process. The surrender piece is even more important and also more profound. Usually, there is a single moment in the labor process where you can see surrender come into the room. I used to say that I would cry twice at every birth. The first is when the baby is born, but the other is when the mom lets go and just trusts her body."

"Trusts her body." That phrase alone is enough to bring tears to my eyes.

Beyond childbirth, when we trust our bodies to tell us about hunger and fullness, exhaustion and energy, they communicate everything we could ever need to know about how to survive and how to thrive.

We don't think of patience or surrender as harbingers of power, but they are at the root of a kind of power women possess that men frequently do not. These two insurgent qualities can be used to subvert the jackasses trying to keep us quiet. Stealth. We may not always be able to out-muscle brutes abusing their positions of power, but we can, without a doubt, out-maneuver them. Like pythons lying in wait for prey to cross our paths, we can watch and wait with pristine patience, preserving our energy for the moment when they get so drunk with power that they stumble. When that happens we will be ready to take them down with all of the imagination, intelligence, endurance, and organizational know-how we have marshaled in the meantime.

This shift is already happening, and our status and our country will never be the same.

Patience is not a lack of action. It's a tactical technique, employed by every woman who ever waited for the right moment to spring a weekend renovation project on her partner or a trip to the Valley of the Gods—or whatever her poison. Patience and preparation come naturally to many of us. I'm generalizing, of course, but it's a truth I witness all around me. Women can see the long game. We can pass the ball from one expert set of hands to the next and make it to the end zone, but *it does take a village*. We care about our communities, so we tend to carry the wonderful but considerable weight of our families' and friends' needs on our backs. None of us can do it alone, but if each of us steps up when our particular set of skills is needed, we will accomplish what we set out to do.

But what about surrender? How is surrender useful? It seems passive.

Most intuitive, astute women have the gift of perspective. We understand that strong-arming situations in our lives generally brings a backlash. It creates resistance where there was none before. We know it from dieting. We know it from wrangling toddlers, teenagers, lovers, bosses, employees, and aging parents into doing what needs to be done. We know how to duck and dodge with the ebb and flow of our circumstances, and if we're smart, we have learned how to turn around and move with the force of the wind at our backs. At our best, we are agile, flexible, and undeterred in the face of adversity.

When we talk about surrender, we are not talking about giving in to the status quo, we're talking about allowing the current state of affairs to wash over us without exhausting us. We're talking about being physically and psychologically prepared to dive into the obscene, oil-slicked mess of gender biases; ready to subvert condescending, power-hungry authority figures who are standing ramrod straight, defensive, with their feet sunk stubbornly in the oily, muddy water. We're talking about having the fortitude to put on our swimsuits, step down into that water, and duck under the surface to take turns digging a sinkhole for ignorant bullies to slip quietly into the deep.

We need our strength for the moments when we will have to dig with all of our heavenly might to uproot the foundation of a system that has subjugated too many human beings for too long. We are capable of extraordinary accomplishments, but we undermine our progress every time we trash ourselves based on how we look.

We can change our status in society, but we'll be standing in quicksand if we don't start where it all begins—with appreciation for our bodies as trustworthy reflections of our heritage and life experiences. Surrender to that inheritance can bring incredible relief and a startling desire to take care of the living, breathing bodies that we have.

Appreciation for our physical bodies is the wildest form of disobedience and the most fundamental step we can take to break free from the chains that bind us.

When I asked Ami why she became a midwife, she told me, "I spent years trying to get out of my body, doing drugs, and doing all of these spiritual practices. I got really sick of this idea of ascension, this whole patriarchal notion that we can 'rise above' and 'get out of,' and I was like, you know what? I love the Earth. I want to celebrate the muck and the blood and the shit of life. This is who we are, and I'm not going to spend my time up there. I want to be right down here in it."

She quoted another midwife saying, "'Birth is supposed to be intense, and you could say it is even supposed to be painful, but it should never mean suffering.' As soon as there is suffering, we need to change the situation. If we've moved into the realm of suffering, we need to make it stop."

Ladies, we are suffering. I can tell you after fifteen years as a personal trainer who has witnessed more suffering than I care to remember that we are stuffed and starving at the same time. Weakened by poor body image, exhausted by shouldering the shit-show on the evening news and trying to solve all of the problems all at once, we sabotage our own agendas. There is a lot we can't change about the world quickly and without a great deal of effort, but respect for our own bodies is absolutely within our power. The reverberations of that shift reach far and wide. It takes practice not to give a damn about other people's opinions of how your body looks, but it's not as hard as you might think. It's sweet mischief, well worth cultivating.

We are cut off at the neck from bodies that should be sources of power and pleasure, but we can alleviate this particular form of suffering by advocating for each other and recognizing true beauty when we see it in ourselves and in others—rejoicing in unapologetic, unconventional beauty in all of its many forms.

No more diets or weight-loss schemes. No more expectations of what your body should or should not look like according to anyone but you. What matters is how it feels and what it can do. We'll reconsider the questions we're asking. Instead of *Do these pants make me look fat?*, we will ask *Does my body feel stiff and weighed down, or does it feel energized and alive? Have I fed it enough fiber and water today? When was the last time I had a massage or a walk in the park or a good night's sleep? Am I wearing the shitkickers my feet so thoroughly deserve?*

When we make healthy changes, we gain mastery of so many other aspects of our lives. Things fall into place. Something else begins to feel more right: smoother, easier, and better.

None of us will ever be 100 percent clearheaded and filled with boundless vitality, but every single thing we do to contribute to our health bolsters us for the task ahead.

The more freely and honestly we live, the less energy is wasted on worthless endeavors. We cannot and will not fall in line because when we are consumed with controlling our bodies, we are leaking energy, leaching it away one stupid, idiotic weight-loss trend at a time.

There is nothing wrong with wanting to lose weight to feel better, but I can promise you from experience that if you are fully consumed with doing all the things you give a damn about with all the people you love, your body will find its balance. You will begin to crave movement and nourishing food because they stimulate not only your body but your imagination as well. The guilt cycle of starve-and-binge will cease, and the weight that plagues you will either fall away or begin to feel wholly natural.

We are trying to hold on to air, people, but we will never get a hold of it. When times are scary and we feel like we're losing ground, the best and only thing we can do is open our lungs to the coming and going of breath, to oxygenate our muscles and bring that vital life force to our brains.

• • •

Let's make a choice to surrender to the present reality—right now, today—in our bodies and in the body politic. Let the insecurity of not knowing what's coming next and the horror of a societal reality steeped in ignorance and hate swirl around us. It's happening, and it sucks. We're doing everything we can to help in every way we can, except taking care of our well-being. Too often, we forget that part.

Our task is clear: to liberate and empower our bodies so that we can liberate and empower our lives.

Freedom lies in the choice to take care of ourselves, moving through and beyond pain, stress, and anxiety. Crack your knuckles and lick your lips. Don't forget to laugh, smile, eat, drink, and rage in the face of disheartening lunacy. It's going to be a hell of a ride, but it's time to take the wheel.

We cannot elicit respect from those in power until we genuinely respect ourselves, recognize our value, and treat our physical bodies with dignity. When we are grounded in and respectful of our own bodies, we can stand firm for what we know is right without wavering, taking blow after blow and holding strong like reeds of grass in an oil-soaked bog.

Wellness is the answer. It is the ultimate form of physical disobedience.

Fill in the Fact

A time I wasted obsessing over my body was _____
_____.

One way I can strengthen my core every day is _____
_____. (*Pssst, plank.*)

I idolize _____ because she _____
_____ even though her body
isn't traditionally "perfect."

I am patiently preparing to change _____
_____ in my life.

Controlling _____ isn't working,
so I'm going to let the situation unfold from here without
wasting my energy.

Appreciation for our physical bodies
is the wildest form of disobedience
and the most fundamental step
we can take to break free from
the chains that bind us.

CHAPTER 3

No Such Thing as Fearlessness

As a progressive in a deeply conservative state, I find myself, way too often, wielding signs to protest legislation on bathroom bills; allowing guns in parks, schools, and bars; defunding of women's health care; or various other draconian laws being proposed in the name of "state's rights" or "religious freedom."

Two weeks after the inauguration of America's forty-fifth president and days after the first "travel ban" was put in place, I was standing with throngs of furious protestors inside the state capitol building on a rope line just before the governor's State of the State address. As legislators passed from meeting rooms to the House Chambers where the speech would be given, I leaned over the red velvet barrier, pointing and chanting "Shame! Shame! Shame!" Directly in front of me, two state troopers stood shoulder to shoulder, making it clear that if I pressed any farther forward, I would be removed.

Senators and representatives streamed past, refusing to engage with the masses of angry constituents.

I screamed frantically at the long line of dark-blue suits with graying hair and finally caught the eye of a red-faced official who paused long enough to observe me like a caged lion. "Lives are at stake!" I yelled. "Lives are at risk because of you! People are suffering! You have blood on your hands!"

He tilted his head, paused, and cracked a cocky smile that said, clear as day, *You're a nut job. Too bad for you, young lady, I have all the power.* He turned on his heel and walked into the Chambers with the swagger of a man unfazed. Foaming at the mouth, I howled along with the chants rising up around me, "No hate. No fear!"

And then the dam of tears broke. They poured over my cheeks and down my blazing hot neck.

My screams were an almost manic expression of the rage and terror saturating my heart. When I cried out to my state representative about blood on his hands, my intention was to speak for people without a voice; to cry out for sensible gun laws to keep deadly weapons out of the hands of criminals and the mentally unstable; and to beg for mercy for my own family. We have preexisting conditions and buy health insurance on the open market.

But the truth was that I didn't know who that legislator was. I didn't know how he had voted on issues I cared about. I was just screaming at whoever had a blank moment to spare for my catharsis. I wasn't screaming at him. I was screaming at the White House and an electorate I could not understand. I was howling at the moon like a wounded mama wolf, unable to save my own child from the darkness of a world where bullies triumph and facts are beside the point.

The president had succeeded in stripping me down and laying me bare, just as he would have me. He left me raw and naked, hemorrhaging venom from every orifice. The tears came from recognizing my powerlessness while, simultaneously, feeling fully supported by a steadfast community of souls at my side, deafening in their protests.

When I got home that evening, I had to step back and check my motives. Rage and fear were justified by the circumstances, but echoes from my past were amplifying them to the point of corrosive panic as flashbacks wormed their way up, hijacking my equilibrium.

There were echoes of a New York City bartender slamming my nineteen-year-old body against an industrial refrigerator at the back of a bar, whipping out his cock, and demanding a hand job in exchange for a piece of bread I had requested to help me sober up so I could find my way back to my dorm in the middle of the night.

There were echoes of a college professor groping me in the darkness of a party in my own apartment, where I managed to dodge his hands, before finding him on top of a nearly unconscious, half-dressed classmate who feared failing his class that semester.

And there were echoes of standing among a circle of young men whom I considered dear friends, all of us in our twenties, and finding my observations interrupted and comprehensively ignored—realizing for the first time that, in their minds, my words didn't matter as much as theirs, no matter how insightful or well-reasoned I was.

In the Capitol Building that night, I chanted, "No hate. No fear," but it was hate and fear that drove me to scream at the closed Chamber doors until my voice broke.

It would be lovely if we could all live free of hatred and fear. I would say we should proceed with fearless abandon toward our new understanding of what beauty looks like and the dedication to health and well-being that has the capacity to change our lives—but that would be dishonest.

There is no such thing as fearlessness. To claim otherwise would require lying to ourselves, and lying breeds weakness. It's empty. It leaves us in danger of collapsing under the slightest bit of pressure, and we're going to need to be more durable than that.

We are all knee deep in fear, as well we should be. We can see how infrequently justice is served, and we shudder at the abundance of anger and violence in the world. There's no question that we are vulnerable, and fear is justified. Life and due process are fragile, but instead of shutting down to those facts or doubling down on liposuction and liquid diets, we will do far better by standing up—stripped of our shiny veneer—to confess the truth.

I am afraid.

I am afraid that I, or someone I love, will be gunned down in a shopping mall by a homegrown madman who can buy a machine gun through the "gun show loophole." I am afraid that planet Earth is breaking down before our eyes with no one in government to defend it. I am afraid that my family and millions of others will be bankrupted by health care costs in the coming years.

And I am enraged.

I am enraged that my son is growing up in a world where masculinity is so often characterized by brutality. I am enraged by Wall Street bankers jetting off to the Caribbean after tanking the economy while young, black men are arrested or shot for wearing the wrong kind of sweatshirts. And I am enraged by my own privilege when I turn on the television to see refugees streaming over borders and starving in makeshift tents.

Denying that fear and rage would be a mistake. We can press the "stay" buttons on our home alarm systems until the beep-beep reassures us, but living freely in this particular world means living with uncertainty. The only thing to do with fear is walk straight into it, abdomens rising and falling, calling it for what it is.

Vulnerability is a hell of a thing to withstand, but when we are raw and stricken with grief as I was on the rope line that night, we are also free—sometimes for the first time in our lives—from the norms of femininity that have constrained us. We're cut loose.

As we watch EPA regulations, civil rights, and international peace fall like raindrops outside our windows, we are abruptly liberated from caring about how our hips and thighs appear. We are free from fretting about the timbre of our voices and the deference of our words. No longer bound by the rules of pretense or decorum, we are gloriously, magnificently unhinged.

If "leadership" thinks we're shrill and unladylike anyway, what do we have to lose? If they value plainspoken, uncensored language and behavior as much as they say they do, let's give them just that. Let's speak plainly in a language they can understand.

• • •

The day before the Republican National Convention in Cleveland, Ohio, in 2016, a photographer named Spencer Tunick and his wife, Kristin Bowler, organized a group of one hundred naked women to descend on the field across the river from the event site for a protest and photo shoot. The women held up mirrors, high above their nude bodies, to reflect the sun onto the convention and to shine a light on women's voices and bodies from all walks of life. In the words of the artists, they were "reflecting the knowledge and wisdom of progressive women and the concept of mother nature onto the convention center."[1]

Interviewed in a short film they made about the protest, one participant said, "Everyone's butts and boobs and bits were all normal and natural, and it was great."

Another said, "If we can accept who we are, accept how we're made, accept each other at the very basic level, I think we're doing great."

And still another, "I felt very liberated . . . and free. That's what America's about, right? Or what it's supposed to be about? Freedom?"

These women were not fearless, but they were bold. Many of them were probably full of fear when the time came to strip off their clothes and stand in an open field in broad daylight and full of fear at the upcoming nomination of a cruel, manhandling brute for president. But they were together, and they were safe. In that safety and through the ability to make their voices heard, they were filled with exhilaration— sweet, audacious liberty.

We all have bumpy "bits." And we all have fear and anger. It's time to let it all hang out. We have too much to do to bother with making sure our bags and shoes match just enough, but not too much. Let's make a collective agreement to let the spinach in our teeth and the toilet paper on our heels be a welcome part of life because, guess what? We eat food and use the bathroom. We are people, not mannequins.

None of us are fearless, but we can carry on if we know that a whole bunch of other people are raging alongside us. Like bike riders in a Tour de France peloton, those of us with the most energy to spare can take the lead, reducing the drag on those behind—so they can keep coming in the slipstream and break out when they are rested up and ready.

It will take endurance to see this through, to prevent fear and rage from eating away at us. Endurance requires pacing, rest, and steady progress. To maintain it, we're going to have to get behind this effort all together and all at once, stripped bare and proud of it.

ALL TOGETHER NOW

In 1963, John F. Kennedy famously said, "A rising tide lifts all boats."

We've been living under the misconception that a small group of women needs to break through the glass ceilings of business and elected office to clear the way for the rest of us, but it hasn't exactly worked out that way. Mary Barra hasn't been able to pull the rest of us up by her coattails just by being CEO of General Motors.

According to the Center for American Women and Politics, on average, women represent 19–25 percent of elected offices from state to national levels.[2] We currently have 20 percent representation in Congress. A study by the Certified Financial Planner Board of Standards tells us that similar percentages hold true for women in financial planning, with their numbers hovering around 23 percent.[3] Women in tech and computer programming fare even worse, with some estimates as low as 8 percent. Google leads the Silicon Valley revolution at a wild and wacky 17 percent of technical employees being women.[4] Female CEOs head up 14 percent of America's companies, and only 4.6 percent of Fortune 500 companies.[5] And women directed just 7 percent of the top 250 films released in 2016.[6]

The numbers for minority women are even more dire, with only 8 percent representation in Congress. And non-white women hold a mere 5 percent of senior-level executive positions in private-sector businesses while they represent over 18 percent of the workforce.[7]

The Center for American Progress reports, "Although women control 80 percent of consumer spending in the United States, they are only 3 percent of creative directors in advertising. Their image onscreen is still created, overwhelmingly, by men. . . . Their 'share of voice'—the average proportion of their representation on op-ed pages and corporate boards, as TV pundits, and in Congress—is just 15 percent. . . . It's now estimated that, at the current rate of change, it will take until 2085 for women to reach parity with men in leadership roles in our country."[8]

2085.

I will be dead. How about you?

Sometimes the world needs inertia. We need it to keep society from running off the rails when politics, law enforcement, and the media collide. We need a big, sluggish colossus of a country to plod along and slow things down enough that everything doesn't implode all at once.

But sometimes we need to heave ho and raise some hell to turn this fucker around.

Every one of us needs to take every opportunity we can to ask why there aren't any women or people of color on the panel. We need to hire female entrepreneurs every chance we get. We need to create scholarships for girls to study robotics and coding. This is a bottom-up operation. When we put the might of our wallets and the bite of ruthless truth telling behind our bid for equality, we will begin to right the ship.

Until recently, we were nags if we "went around complaining" about the fact that there are so few women in leadership, about unequal pay or toxic work environments. But the gears are beginning to groan as we throw our collective weight into changing direction. The #metoo movement of 2017 exposed the horrifying truth that nearly every woman in America has experienced some form of sexual assault or harassment. All at once, we told the truth, calling out men who once wielded enormous power and bringing them to account. It was a remarkable example that there is so much less reason to fear speaking out when we are surrounded by millions of other whip-smart women doing the same.

So why don't more women go into politics or finance? Because the old boys club is annoying. And disheartening. And thick. Because watching our ideas get disregarded before they are stolen and rephrased right in front of our faces isn't the slightest bit rewarding. Because we are passed over for promotions and paid less for our work even when we advocate for ourselves, and because advocating for ourselves is perceived as pushy and combative. We care about quality of life, so a lot of us choose to go into fields where our contributions will be valued and we won't feel like we're fighting a street brawl every day. All of this leaves us with fewer role models and mentors, a chicken-and-egg situation.

The solution isn't for you or me or any of us, alone, to break through to the top. The solution, at least part of it already in evidence, is for all of us to simultaneously start chattering away, making noise whenever and wherever we can, raising our hands and voices, and calling inequality out. We need representation at every level, and not having it is just plain antiquated and indefensible.

Most important, we need to put our money where our mouths are to shop with female-owned businesses at every opportunity and to support female and male candidates running for office whose beliefs align with our own. And, at work, we should expect equal pay and employment in positions both above *and* below us, to make sure young women are in the pipeline, ready to take the reins.

There is a big, wide world outside this here henhouse, and we birthed it. It's our time to have a go at running the show.

Women can be expert planners. We can see the big picture and delegate minutia without missing a beat. We are genetically predisposed to be able to discern and direct the behavior of children. That would seem to come in handy at the moment, considering some of the imbeciles masquerading as leadership, no?

There are swarms of us coming out of neighborhoods nationwide, out of colleges, community centers, schools, nightclubs, religious institutions, gyms, and art studios all over the country to protect the safety of the whole. If we all start "harping" on the same stuff at the same time and don't let up, they'll capitulate just to shut us up, or they'll work themselves into such a tizzy that half of them will end up hospitalized with panic attacks.

But none of this will happen, nothing will change, if we keep apologizing for being short and tall and fat and skinny and smart and human.

SWORD OF PROTECTION

She-Ra, Princess of Power was a cartoon superhero in the 1980s, like a B-level Wonder Woman. She was He-Man's twin sister, a regular woman in daily life who used the power of her "sword of protection" to transform into her superhero alter ego.

According to Wikipedia, "She-Ra is known for her incredible strength. She has been shown to be able to lift not only full-grown men and robots, but also mountain-like rocks and buildings. She is also extremely fast and acrobatic with a series of other abilities . . . such as empathic understanding and communication with animals and healing. . . . Her sword is almost indestructible and able to deflect bolts of energy, both magical and technological. . . . She-Ra is largely nonviolent and only resorts to combat as a last resort. She uses cunning and her wits, often preferring to outsmart her adversaries."[9]

Henceforth, whenever you are overcome by rage or fear, duck beneath your sword of protection. The sword is your chosen contribution, your way of speaking out and reinforcing a much larger movement for equality and human rights. Use it to shield not only your own family and friends but to shelter and defend anyone in need of protection—beyond borders and ideologies, including those who would call you gullible or immoral. These acts of outreach will fortify your broken heart while you ride atop your winged-unicorn, Swift Wind. Delivering this solemn protection as far as the sword may reach will ease the hate and fear that inevitably seep into your flesh and inhabit your mind. (Note: At my house, the part of Swift Wind will be played by a miniature pit bull named Ringo.)

Do not fret over the mammoth responsibility of this task because the sword of protection does not belong to you alone. It belongs to the vast and deep collective of which you are one tiny part—a community of women of every color, along with immigrants, queers, and He-Men who believe that people are equal and worthy of respect, regardless of sex, age, race, or religion. Find your small part of this massive outreach, and utilize it to maintain your balance. But do not take on more than you can manage.

My personal part of the sword is to help each of us find our own unique ways to sustain our physical bodies and *to get those bodies to the polls to VOTE in every election*, both local and national.

We need to be ready when enormous turds from the opposition hit the fan and come flying back in our direction—projectile bullshit that must be smacked down, one pellet of excrement at a time.

We need to go Serena-and-Venus-doubles-match on their asses. And if our arms get tired after five minutes of holding up the sword, we're screwed.

What is your part of the sword? What gets you fired up? What organizations have you considered volunteering with or contributing to but haven't made the leap yet? How are you connected to your local community, and how can you reach out to make a difference face-to-face? If you're not already involved, check out the appendix at the end of the book to get specific ideas for how you can help. You're not just taking a stand for a cause; you're taking a stand for your own body and your long-term health and well-being.

We need to work on behalf of our bodies legislatively, of course, to prevent laws from being passed that will strip us of our autonomy, but we also urgently need to work on our bodies' behalfs to reinforce them, thereby boosting our spirits and releasing ourselves from distorted standards of beauty and value.

We need our strength. We need our bodies. We must give them the respect they deserve, the nourishment they need, and the physical movement they crave.

Sikh-American civil rights advocate Valarie Kaur gave a speech in front of a congregation at Metropolitan African Methodist Episcopal Church in Washington, DC, on New Year's Eve, December 2016. I call it a speech, but it was more than that. It was an outcry.

"Black bodies are still seen as criminal," she said, "brown bodies are still seen as illegal, trans bodies are still seen as immoral, indigenous bodies are still seen as savage, the bodies of women and girls seen as someone else's property, and when we see these bodies not as brothers and sisters, then it becomes easier to bully them, to rape them, to allow policies that neglect them, that incarcerate them, that kill them. . . . The future is dark . . . but on this watch night . . . the mother in me asks, 'What if?' What if this darkness is not the darkness of the tomb but the darkness of the womb? What if our America is not a country that is dead, but a country that is waiting to be born? . . . What if this is our nation's great transition?"

● ● ●

A rising tide lifts all boats. We are the tide. When we strengthen our communities, we strengthen ourselves, and when we strengthen ourselves, we strengthen our communities.

The challenges we face are daunting, but the work of supporting our own well-being and the well-being of those around us is there to set us free, right away, any time we want it.

Taking care of our health is not a chore. It's one of the best parts of being alive. It demands magnifying our bodies, stretching and dancing and eating beautiful, sweet, spicy, whole, and filling food.

When disgusting, absurd political stories weigh us down and we watch our neighbors falling victim to inhumane policies, we have to move. Sword of protection activate! It's the only way to survive this foolishness.

Fill in the Fact

I am pissed off about _____
_____.

And also about _____
_____.

I'm afraid that _____
_____.

I am 100 percent ready to "harp" about _____
_____.

My sword/contribution protects _____
_____.

A group I've been curious about supporting is _____
_____.

After spending a few hours helping _____,
I feel _____.

Vulnerability is a hell of a thing to withstand, but when we are raw and stricken with grief, we are also free—sometimes for the first time in our lives—from the norms of femininity that have constrained us. We're cut loose.

PART 2

BODY UNLEASHED

CHAPTER 4

Bodies Don't Lie

We all know how it feels to be "off," to have recurring nausea or headaches. *I don't feel right. I'm bloated. I'm queasy. My back hurts.* Messages like this flow through our bodies every day. I imagine these sensations like tiny mice, running around on a field in the packed football stadium, wearing feather boas and carnival hats, jumping up and down to get our attention. They're doing everything they can, squeaking with all their might, but they haven't got a shot in hell at being heard.

Illnesses, aches, and pains nag at us all the time. As a trainer, I hear about them every day, and the same old complaints can persist for years or even decades. Sometimes they go away on their own, but dismissed or ignored, many get worse over time. In response, we do everything we can to dodge the symptoms, to manage or numb the discomfort.

If we're in pain, we tell ourselves that we're imagining it, that it will pass, and we turn a blind eye. Or, alternately, we project the worst possible outcome, assume it will last forever, and give up entirely in exchange for opioids or dark rooms with the blinds drawn. If we are out of shape and unhappy with how we look and feel, we set explicit goals for how our bodies should appear and direct them to comply—even if the diet plan is miserable and the workouts are unsustainable. And if our bodies don't respond to these commands in the ways we want, we shut them down with booze, pills, pizza, or screen time.

We are disembodied and reprimanding everything below the collarbone. We lecture our bodies all the time about how they should look and behave but don't spend nearly enough time listening to them. Our bodies are our greatest teachers. The ability to heed what they are telling us before unhealthy conditions become chronic and insurmountable is the most important tool we can cultivate to live better, lighter, and more effectively.

Stress slides through our veins like magma through a volcano. Too much sugar or alcohol poisons our blood. You can feel the symptoms of bad nutrition or too much time at work as you drift off to sleep or as you lay awake dreading the ticking of the clock. Crappy goes to bed with you and spends the night.

A hangover is a gift from the overindulgence gods to let you know that you've gone too far. "Maybe stick to one or two drinks next time," it says, but do you listen? A sore back tells you that you could probably use some stretching and strengthening, but a steady drumbeat of muted grunting and a daily dose of Alleve are easier to wrap your head around.

Our bodies communicate quite clearly when it's time to take another approach, but we are deaf and blind, distracted by the shiny lights and thunderous roar of the action all around us.

IGNORING THE SQUEAKS

When finishing the manuscript for my first book, I developed a rash under my right boob, which I wrongly assumed to be yeast. I was at the beach and thought my wet bathing suit was to blame. By the time I self-medicated with an expired fluconazole pill and waited a few days for it not to work, the rash grew painful and reached around to my back as well. When I made it home and to the doctor, she told me I didn't have a yeast infection. I had shingles. Stunned, I responded, "But I'm not a seventy-year-old man! I can't have shingles. I'm not even forty yet!"

"Yes," she said, "you can. All it takes is previous exposure to chicken pox and a weakened immune system. Have you been stressed out lately?"

Ummmm.

There were many alarm bells leading up to this revelation. I wasn't sleeping. I was tired all the time. I was craving sweets and fried food. My neck hurt. My digestion wasn't right. I hadn't had a diet soda in years, but out of nowhere, those caramel bubbles were tempting again.

My mice were making a ruckus, and I was running all over the football field in the middle of the game, trying to chase them down while dodging human cannonballs the size of tanker trucks: My dad had cancer. My grandma was forgetting which of her adult children was married to whom. My son was three years old, sweet but exhausting. My training business was too busy to handle—and I had this big dream unfolding. I was writing a book! "Cadillac problem," my husband would say, but could I actually write it and write it well? Could I do it by the deadline? As the due date tapped at my back door, *squeak, squeak*, went the mice.

I did get to the deadline with a beautiful manuscript in hand and spent a few months afterward reconnecting with my sanity in order to manage the heavier issues still swirling. But the following year when I got distracted again and stopped doing the powerful work to ease my stress level—funny thing—out of nowhere my shoulder went bad. Like really bad.

Being the smart aleck that I am, I decided—again—to treat it myself. I knew how to rest and ice and stretch and strengthen. I'm an expert, right? When that didn't work and I was no longer able to reach for the seat belt in my car, I went for a month of physical therapy and kept the exercises up dutifully for another six months. Still in pain and losing sleep at night, I finally went to an orthopedist, the first of many steps to get my mobility back. Clearly, I wasn't doing a very good job of listening.

HEEDING THE CALL

Our bodies have something to say. They are talking to us all the time. But if we aren't listening, if we're running the show from way up in our heads and disregarding the messages from below, we're likely to end up with frozen shoulder, digestive issues, plantar fasciitis, food addiction, shingles, or whatever other somatic symptoms our bodies can throw at us to get our attention.

It's a slippery slope. When our bodies cry out with aches and pains, or for simple touch or movement, if we don't heed the call, we hover a long way from healing.

I take care of people's bodies for a living. I'm the "pro" in the gym all day, helping my clients figure out how best to heal, but while I was distracted, trying to hear their messages and ignoring my own, my shoulder congealed into hardened cheese.

Sure, I went to physical therapy and did the exercises they assigned, but I also continued to lift heavy weights and hand them at awkward angles to my clients all day. I thought about going to acupuncture but never could find the time or money. I knew all kinds of treatments I should be trying, but didn't make it a priority to get them done.

As I sit here, writing this passage, I am humbled by pain. The squeak has become a blaring siren. I wasn't listening. It didn't have to be this way, but here I am. Now I have to commit to healing like my life depends on it—because it does. My health and happiness depend on it. I can't do anything without it hurting, and that's not acceptable.

So as we launch into this part of the book where we're talking about various ways to get our bodies in balance, please know that none of it is coming from up on a soapbox. I'm in this process with you, trying to heal my own thing. We'll dive in to everything from how we feed and strengthen our bodies to how we dress and rest them. We need options, lots of them, and we have to keep looking until we find some that work for each of us—with our unique bodies, ailments, and proclivities.

I'll be working on the shoulder situation as I write and will let you know in the end how it goes. No outcome is guaranteed. Bodies aren't math problems with definitive answers. They are delicate ecosystems that are constantly in the process of mending themselves, but they need as much reinforcement as they can get.

Why is it so difficult to support that natural equilibrium? Why is it so hard to remember to take care of ourselves? Because chips are delicious, and TV is distracting. Pills take the edge off, and capitulating to an injury feels safer than working to overcome it. Quick fixes are extremely seductive—until we wake up five years later and realize we are still in exactly the same situation, with exactly the same underlying conditions, plus fifteen pounds and a sore knee.

Give your mice a microphone by answering a few straightforward questions:

- Do you have any unexplained aches and pains hanging around?
- What about skin conditions, hair loss, or stomach problems?
- Are you sleeping better or worse than you used to?
- Are you more forgetful, distracted, or irritable?
- Do you have cravings for food or behaviors that make you feel worse afterward?
- Is there a time of day when fatigue, depression, or anxiety regularly show up?
- Was there a clear onset of these symptoms or did they sneak up on you over time?

Finding solutions to these problems is a long and winding road. There will be some suggestions in later chapters, but the most straightforward advice I can give you is this:

1. Hear your body—and take note of what it is telling you. On paper. On your phone. On a calendar. What is it telling you and when?
2. Live consciously with the effects of the messages your body is sending for a week or a month or a year. Let yourself off the hook for a little while—free of guilt or judgment—so you can understand and appreciate the real impact they are having on your life and body. This awareness is crucial to solidify your motivation.
3. Find *small, manageable* behavioral changes to give the mice what they are asking for. Stick to them, and give yourself enough time to feel the payoff—several months or more.

I have worked with people from ages sixteen to ninety-two and from one hundred to four hundred pounds, all of whom were looking for a healthier relationship with their bodies. Sometimes dramatic changes are either medically necessary or readily implemented for those who have hit the wall and are ready for a radically different way of life. But, for most people, small changes are a lot more likely to stick, and they have a much more profound impact than you might imagine.

There are countless ways to support your health and well-being. You just need to grab hold of them, whenever you get the chance, to get a little stronger each day, rather than weaker. I know it sounds simplistic. It's hard to believe that small actions make much of a difference, but the fact is they make all the difference.

Try being a health opportunist, and watch what happens.

Snag every opportunity to walk up a flight of stairs; help put away chairs after a community meeting; grab a snack from the fruit bowl every afternoon before your energy drops; turn off the TV when there's nothing good on and organize your closet instead; or schedule a walking meeting rather than sitting at a coffee shop. These small adaptations shape the ways our bodies function over time. They sprout new connections in our brains that encourage more movement, more healthy food, and more social and professional connections. Following through on this stuff takes relatively little effort. It's a no-brainer, but it does require a nudge. It requires an open mind and willingness to make a different choice than you would on autopilot.

• • •

By the time I saw a specialist for my shoulder, it was so far gone that the doctor had to shoot me up with cortisone—straight to the joint—while I did a dead-on imitation of Wile E. Coyote at the moment he steps off the cliff. I'd prefer never to experience that again. From here, the progress is up to me. Doc says priority #1 is getting my range of motion back. It's slow going, and the stretches burn like fire. As I inch my way deeper into each position, I shut my eyes and release my gut. I talk to the muscles like they are sentient beings. *Let's have a chat, deltoid. Let go please. It's safe. I know you're trying to protect the joint, but it's okay. Just give me another centimeter, one more, and hold right there.* Breathe.

The master plan is to stretch multiple times a day; ice at night; get massage and acupuncture; increase anti-inflammatory foods in my diet and decrease inflammatory ones; and take over-the-counter pain killers at night as needed.

Sticking with a routine like this might be difficult if I approach it the way I used to look at fitness. *This sucks! It's a hassle! An imposition! It's robbing me of my freedom!* But over time, I have realized—like a frying pan to the head—that, no, doing what's right for my body is not robbing me of my freedom.

The *pain* is robbing me of my freedom. The *sugar addiction* is robbing me of my freedom, and the *lack of energy* is robbing me of my freedom.

The more disconnected my body becomes from health and vitality, the fewer autonomous choices I am able to make. So when I work to reach one inch higher, one inch closer to normal with the arm I haven't straightened in nearly a year, it will be for so much more than my own remedial care. It will be explicitly for my freedom and for everything I care about. It will be for the many more times I expect to have to hold up signs to express my dismay at arts programs or educational funding being slashed. It will be for wrangling my dog and high-fiving my kid. And it will be in defiance of the belief that women are weak and that our shoulders are primarily for showing off spaghetti straps.

Shoulders are for lifting. They are for swinging and embracing, and I want all of those abilities back in spades.

YOUR NERVOUS SYSTEM IS THE CENTER OF YOUR UNIVERSE

The injuries, diseases, and destructive habits that we struggle with frequently start out small. They originate in one part of the body and are fueled by a bad habit or two, but they have a tendency to spread. Once you've got a twisted ankle, your hip goes weird, which causes you to hold your posture funny, which messes with your back. Over time, the pain becomes distracting, amplifying it all the more and beginning a snowball effect. The same applies for weight loss and unhealthy eating. You feel tired so you eat junk to boost your energy. The junk makes you feel guilty, defeated, and lethargic again, so you eat some more. Here we go round the mulberry bush.

This snowball effect is a real physiological thing called central sensitization. According to Tracy Jackson, MD, a chronic pain physician at Vanderbilt University and founder of Relief Retreats,[1] "Central sensitization occurs when the central nervous system (the brain and spinal cord) receives intense or ongoing input. This causes these nerves to 'wind up' and become more sensitive. If the brain receives a large signal or an ongoing barrage of signals that the body is not safe (i.e. pain from a broken bone, a 'fight or flight' surge from fear/anxiety, etc.), the brain dials up the sensitivity, to remind the body to stay on high alert.

"For example, if a signal like nausea from anxiety is persistent, it can become full-blown irritable bowel syndrome," she said. "The bowel becomes more sensitive to every pang of fear, and these ongoing bowel symptoms produce more anxiety. The vicious cycle ensues, and then, all of a sudden a 'normal' pain from exercise can become debilitating, chronic back pain. It doesn't matter which of these things occurs first (back pain, knee pain, abdominal pain, anxiety, trauma, stress, insomnia). If the initial signal is intense or ongoing enough, everything gets revved up, so people stop moving and try to protect themselves from what feels like a saber-toothed tiger."

The systems of the body all work together. The skeletal, circulatory, respiratory, digestive, reproductive, and excretory systems (among others) all communicate, and the nervous system connects with them all. The nervous system perceives, informs, and responds to both your internal and external experiences of being alive. It can keep everything moving smoothly, or—as Dr. Jackson described above—it can overreact and heighten our experience of pain or suffering. The nervous system regulates heart rate and respiration; it allows us to recognize sensations like touch, taste, and smell; and it receives and responds to alarm bells telling us *NUCLEAR WAR IS A BAD IDEA. VERY. BAD. IDEA. PANIC. MUST DO SOMETHING!*

Our mental and emotional states impact our physical well-being, and the other way around. And, of course, stress heightens all of it.

When you're stressed, one or more of the following are likely to happen to your body:

- Heart rate goes up.
- Muscles tense and get achy and stiff.
- Stomach turns, causing indigestion, heartburn, constipation, or diarrhea.
- Immune system suffers, causing more raunchy colds.
- Sleep suffers.
- Appetite goes through the roof or disappears.
- Nutrition and energy suffer.
- Sex life withers.

If you're trying to make a presentation at work or deal with soccer practice, a dentist appointment, a gymnastics meet, dinner, and an unexpected visit from your relatives at the same time—and you only slept three hours last night because your foot keeps cramping up and the rent is due and you can't remember the last time you got laid—your day is pretty much shot. And your nervous system has gone apeshit bananas.

By the time you find yourself in a situation like that, every system in your body is on edge, and trying to isolate ailments or parts of the body is futile.

If you've got an acute situation that is directly treatable, such as a broken bone or a hormone imbalance that needs correcting, of course, you go to the doctor and take care of it as needed. But if messages from multiple mice are blending into a cacophony of atonal squeaks and shrieks, you need a kumbaya moment with all the body parts at once. You need to soothe the whole system.

Trying to break damaging habits (such as stress eating, shopping too much, or biting your nails) when your nervous system is on fire is about as pointless as trying to increase women's representation in Congress by carving the faces of Gloria Steinem and Susan B. Anthony into the rock face of Stone Mountain, Georgia, before the authorities come after you with tear gas and handcuffs. Not happening. But if you can pay attention to what is happening system-wide in your body and mind (and the circumstances triggering the stress)—and if you can respond with steady, proactive, holistic care—most of the time, you can bring your body back into balance before the whole apparatus spins out of control.

HEALING THE BODY TO HEAL THE MIND

If you care about feeling stronger, if you want to stop the brain-barf that repeatedly tells you that you're unworthy, or if you hope to boost your energy for what you love to do, your body is quite literally the path to freedom. It is the vehicle that will carry you to opportunities you might have believed were out of reach. And relieving your body of stress is the most important thing you can do to liberate your inner renegade.

People endure unimaginable stress. When I think about how human bodies survive famine and carpet bombing and single parenthood, I am in awe. People survive, but the strain burns—physically. The barrage takes a toll on our bodies. I wish the stinging could stop somehow, for all of us. I wish it would come to an end and all would be peaceful in the world, but that's not likely to happen. And even if it did, it wouldn't be life. It would be a weird limbo state of nonliving.

There's no way around uncertainty and pain, but there is a lot we can do to relieve our nerves and muscles. Some of it costs money. If you can afford to get the treatment you need, don't ever feel like it's a waste. It's the furthest thing from it. But if you can't afford expensive therapies, there are still lots of options, and the free ones are often the best ones anyway. See Chapter 7 for information on a few specific treatments that might be fun to try whether or not you have cash to spare.

Talk therapy can help, with a professional or even with a trusted friend. Airing out your worries by speaking truth to another human being is a well-established way of dealing with depression and anxiety, and increasingly, therapists are learning that addressing the body's *physical* symptoms of stress can be an essential piece of the puzzle.

We can read books about personal transformation all day. We can dig up our pasts in search of explanations. We can take lessons from others and listen to enlightening stories of catharsis and redemption. All of these methods help. All of them are valuable, but without our bodies along for the ride, we're stuck.

When it comes to the shadows of our consciousness—the impulses and decades-old beliefs that drive destructive behaviors and preventable chronic conditions—our bodies are immediate resources for healing.

In an interview with Krista Tippett on NPR's *On Being*, the medical director of the Trauma Center at the Justice Resource Institute, Bessel van der Kolk, said, "You secrete stress hormones in order to give you the energy to cope under extreme situations . . . to stay up all night with your sick kid or to shovel snow in Minnesota and Boston and stuff like that. What goes wrong is, if you're kept from using your stress hormones, if somebody holds you down, if somebody keeps you imprisoned, the stress hormones keep going up, but you cannot discharge [them] with action. Then the stress hormones really start wreaking havoc with your own internal system. But as long as you move, you are going to be fine. As we know, after these hurricanes and these terrible things, people get very active. They like to help; they like to do things, and they enjoy doing it because it discharges their energy. . . . We are using our natural system, basically. We're not only healing; we're coping."[2]

The stress that dogs you in your life-at-large is also defeating your ability to heal an old injury or achieve a healthy weight, which is getting in the way of everything else. The ex who screwed you over, the boss who undervalues your work, the food cravings you can't shake, the roommate who drives you nuts, the wretched evening news, they are all messing with your health. Some of them you might be able to change; some of them you might not, at least not right away. But what you can do, right now, is find a few ways to alleviate the physical symptoms of those stressors.

Send out a giant middle finger to all of it. Allow yourself to be pissed about it and brokenhearted. Find an empty field to stand in, and scream your guts out. And then wrap yourself up in the cradle of a warm bath or a favorite old T-shirt and jeans before heading out for your daily dose of opportunism: fresh air, exercise, real food, and purposeful acts of kindness.

Your body is trying to tell you something when you are stressed out, in pain, or eating for no reason in the middle of the night.

When you have listened to the mice for long enough and heard the messages your body is trying to send, if pain or stress or an infuriatingly frustrating bad habit surfaces, meet it with physical disobedience.

Move. It will heal you.

- When you are exhausted from sitting behind a desk all day clicking on noxious internet commentary, ready to withdraw into the hinterland of your psyche with a solid dose of Kung Pao and booze before passing out with a box of cookies by the couch—put on your sneakers and walk or drive to a designated location that makes your shoulders drop. Roll your head around to loosen your neck. Stand up straight, and clasp your hands behind your back with the wrong pinky clasped on top. Roll open your chest, and pull your shoulder blades together like they are bound by a thick rubber band. Defy close-mindedness and cruelty by opening your heart and engaging your body. They can't have it. It belongs to you.
- When you are exhausted from a long, overly eventful day and you think you should return some

emails and weed your pitiful flower bed and start a load of laundry—grab a blanket instead, and a pillow, and lay down on the couch. Shut your eyes, and rest. Do nothing at all, even if only for ten minutes, even if there are small children or multiple pets yammering in all directions. Defy the expectation that you must be ON all the time in order to be an effective, responsible person. Give yourself ten minutes. They can't have it. It belongs to you.

- When your in-laws come to visit and start criticizing the storage methods in your kitchen cabinets—leave the Tupperware drawer in a particularly fabulous state of upheaval for their arrival and enthusiastically invite anyone who has a problem with it to have a go at organizing it. When they return the following year to find it back in its natural state, inform them that they are welcome to organize it each time they visit, but, in the interim, the kitchen is yours. They can't have it. It belongs to you.

- And when rage and fear begin to overtake your stability—rage right back with a run or a rally, a yoga class or a clothing swap, a night out dancing with friends or a casserole assembly line aimed at feeding every family you can think of who might be feeling broke and strung out. Do anything except eat your feelings and let your muscles gelatinize. You have the power to nurture your body instead of abusing it. They can't have that power. It belongs to you.

• • •

Identify the negative ways you are succumbing to stress, and find direct, proactive ways to defy it—ways that heal and strengthen your body and mind.

I have seen this approach work wonders with my clients over the years. One of them, Abby, is a lighthearted person by nature. She works in city planning. It's not glamorous, but her job is crucial for those of us who love our sidewalks and neighborhoods. She is underpaid and overworked. She is a reluctant activist when she can manage it and a musical theater nerd whenever shows pass through town. She believes in people and kindness and baking for the common good. She is single in her early forties and the truest kind of friend. She carries more weight on her body than she would like but has been moving steadily toward a different kind of appreciation for what "healthy" might look and feel like for her.

Abby came in for a session a few months ago in pieces. There was shock on her face and fear in her body. She was sick that afternoon with a lingering cough, and her house had been broken into the night before for the *third* time. It was ransacked and emptied of valuable possessions. She was stripped of a sense of safety in her home, and the news bombarding both of us raged with missile launches, health care wars, and school shootings. It was too much. She could barely breathe.

My gym is a quiet place, a sunroom off the back of my house. The floor is made of soft, thick rubber, and the walls are painted Aqua Pura, a shade of watery-blue. We lay down flat on our backs on the floor and reached as far as our arms and legs could stretch. We breathed in and out and waited for our insides to unclench. We hugged our knees and rocked from side-to-side before allowing them to fall, bent to one side with our arms spread out in the shape of a T. We twisted to the left and then to the right, wringing out all the things we could not change. When she had steadied herself, we rose to plank until our arms shook and abdomens burned, jolting our lungs and hearts back to life. We moved through a series of exercises and, in the end, collapsed into child's pose to release our backs and rest.

When we were done, we exchanged a glance that said, *I can't even believe this shit, but press on sister*—and we established that she needed to get the hell out of that house, for good. We raised a cool glass of water to feeling better, just for a minute, and to knowing we had the power to shape more loose and long minutes whenever we felt like it.

• • •

We don't have to live in constant reaction to whack-a-mole aches and pains. We can be proactive. If the world keeps bringing ups and downs (which it always will), our job is to bring a deluge of good practices, to keep our bodies in good working order so we're ready for whatever comes next.

To pull that off, we need to listen for the faint squeaks and make our tiny mice a priority, scooping them up with gentle hands to put them in happy, hamster-wheel worlds where they can get their groove on: running off energy, drinking enough water, resting peacefully, and playing with their friends.

Mayday. Something is wrong. We have to stop talking and start listening. When our bodies hurt or yearn to be loaded up with carbs and alcohol to take the edge off, it's time to pay attention.

I am learning, finally, to pay attention.

GIVE IT A BREAK

Standing in a darkened bar last week, I was listening to my friend Sally play music up onstage.[3] My eyes were closed. Another friend was dancing next to me with her heels in one hand and her drink in the other. It was late, and my body was still. I wondered if Sally could see me, if she would wonder why I wasn't dancing, but the feeling washing over me was exquisite just as it was. If I moved, I was afraid it would slip away. I could feel the rhythm of the bass pulsing through me. My chest was open. My jaw was loose. I didn't need another sip of wine. I could feel the naked shape of my hips and abdomen under my clothes and paused with my attention there. I spent so many years in bars just like this, distracted by my body in a different way—my jeans and shirt clinging too tight in all the wrong places. But not tonight. To-night my body was my own, without discomfort or apology.

I made reliable peace with my body a while back, but I rarely take the time to notice what that actually means, how different music feels when I can absorb it rather than trying to shape it into an accessory for my next pose, the most flattering angle.

That night in the bar was sublime. Music and friends were there, and my body was there, present and accounted for. I rolled my head around to stretch my neck and placed a hand on my faulty shoulder. If I could learn to love, so thoroughly, this body that I used to despise, I could find the endurance to nurse my broken wing back to good health. It is part of me, and it is in need of rescue. I will not leave it behind.

● ● ●

Putting down the dietary and fitness weapons you've deployed against your body for so many years and letting go of the mechanisms you've used to keep it under control can be scary, but those tools haven't kept you safe. They've made you crazy. The only way to start listening is to be aware of your body just as it is, however broken or whole. The safest way to take care of it is to hear what it is telling you and, when you're ready, push it gently out of its comfort zone.

You can lie flat on your back or hold a wobbly plank. You can stand in a bar and dance or not dance. You can slide into a bath or hike Kili-manjaro. I've got your back, and everyone else reading this book does, too.

What's not safe is expecting perfection from yourself or anyone else or expecting validation of your body to come from someone else's opinion of it. Lovers are notoriously unreliable, and haters who want to tell you what your body is supposed to look like are in no position to judge. Let their hatred eat away at their own flesh, not yours.

• • •

Talking with a friend of mine, Paige de Wees, a Buddhist hospital chaplain in St. Paul, Minnesota, I asked how she approaches her own self-care in what is presumably a very challenging profession. With a smile, she responded, "If I don't plug in my phone, it's going to die."

Your body is disruptive and loud. Let it be. Listen to it closely, and plug it back in as often as you can, in as many ways as you can, to recharge and get even louder and more disruptive with each passing day.

Your body is telling you when something is wrong. Don't cut it off or shut it down. Take heed of the tiny squeaks and respond in kind.

◇◇

Fill in the Fact

My _____ hurts.

I have tried to heal it by _____
_____.

This makes it worse: _____
_____.

This makes it better: _____
_____.

I have not tried _____
but am curious to see if it might help.

I think my body is trying to tell me that _____

_____.

One specific way I can respond to that message is _____

_____.

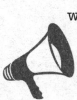

Identify the negative ways you
are succumbing to stress, and find
ways to defy it—ways that heal and
strengthen your body and mind.

CHAPTER 5

Exercise

Let's get real about one thing before going any further: Exercise, by itself, will not make you lose a bunch of weight. For too long, the vast majority of us have associated exercise with the end goal of weight loss. This seemingly reasonable assumption is a distortion of the truth that perpetuates a frustrating cycle and blinds us to the many other benefits of challenging our bodies.

As a personal trainer, it is not in my self-interest to tell you this, but it's the truth, borne out by a ton of scientific research.[1] Anyone who tries to sell you on exercise as a weight-loss method without regard to what you're eating and how you're spending your downtime is either uninformed or trying to put one over on you.

Exercise can help you lose a little weight (as in a few pounds), and it can certainly help you keep it off, but without changing something permanent about the way you eat and how much you move each day when you're *not* working out, exercise won't magically turn you into your skinny-self, no matter how hard you work at the gym.

When we exercise more, our brains prompt us to eat more to fuel the extra effort and rest more to recover. Have you ever trained for a 10K or joined a boot camp only to discover that you don't lose a pound? Your strength and endurance go up. You have more energy, but the scale doesn't budge. That's because your body is fighting to maintain the status quo. This makes evolutionary sense. When we burn a lot of calories, our bodies strive to conserve as much energy as possible. We also become ravenous in an attempt to replace the calories spent.

Ever since leotards and legwarmers hit the scene in the early 1980s, the story we have been told is that exercise will make you thin. It won't. It certainly makes you strong, but it also makes you hungry.

So that sucks. We all thought that if we just got off the couch and busted our butts for thirty to sixty minutes a day, we would drop the extra pounds. Unfortunately, it doesn't work that way, and that myth has done a lot of damage. It's one of many contributors to the obesity epidemic. We believe exercise is the magic bullet, so we sweat as hard as we can. But when it doesn't make a difference on the scale, we get frustrated and give up. We end up back on our butts feeling like failures and turn to distracted eating to make ourselves feel better. I used to chase the fantasy of exercise for weight loss, too, and it destroyed my confidence. It made me feel inadequate and weak, but once I understood what exercise is actually *for* and placed the right expectations on it, everything changed.

If we get our heads in the right place, we can transform the reasons we exercise. We can remove the guilt cycle associated with not working out hard enough and start moving on purpose: to reduce our pain and power our ambitions.

Weight loss aside, exercise is one of the best things you can do for your peace of mind, your relationships, and possibly even for your paycheck. It will boost your strength, confidence, mood, and focus. It will reduce your odds of insomnia, depression, stroke, heart attack, high blood pressure, diabetes, and dementia. It will increase your muscle mass, bone density, metabolism, memory, and sex drive. Together, all of these improvements increase your sense of well-being, which impacts everything you do. With those changes in place, eating well gets easier and permanent weight loss becomes more plausible because you're not overtaxing your body and exhausting your willpower.

Another upside? Regular exercise will make you more beautiful—in the truest sense—not necessarily because you're thinner but because it stimulates your circulatory system. It pumps nutrient-rich blood throughout your body and rejuvenates your skin. Exercise improves your posture and turns the lights on in your brain. People can see the difference in your eyes and in the way you carry yourself when you're rooted joyfully in your body.

Exercise is for accessing power, not for losing weight. By moving, we are waking our bodies up, not making them surrender.

Also, please scrap the concept of "No pain, no gain." You do not need to hurt yourself to get healthy. If you need a catch phrase, "No action, no traction" is more like it. You need to move and stretch—not so that you can get smaller, but so that you can claim your space.

Movement is life-giving, and that's the point.

If you exercise for the wrong reasons and in ways you hate, the effort will suck you dry. If you exercise for the right reasons and in ways you love, it will invigorate you—and you might be surprised what "exercise" can look like if you allow yourself a little space to redefine it.

EXERCISE DOESN'T HAVE TO MEAN SLAVING AWAY AT THE GYM

Laurie Green is the founder of SAFPAW, the Southern Alliance for People and Animal Welfare, an organization that helps homeless communities and the pets that keep them warm and connected on the streets.[2] For the past twenty-two years, Laurie has been in the field, several times a week, hauling supplies to tent cities and homeless camps tucked away beneath underpasses and deep in the woods. She transports animals every Wednesday from the camps to spay/neuter clinics and brings them back to their owners the following day when the procedures are done. She supplies regular vet care and food for the pets as well.

For the people, many of whom she has known personally for decades, she brings fresh water, food, tents, tarps, heaters, propane, sleeping bags, bug spray, feminine products, and socks. She also helps them track down their birth certificates and social security cards so they can attain state IDs. You and I might not think twice about the importance of these records, but it's essentially impossible to find a job or get an apartment without basic identification.

When she's not out on the streets, Laurie is running Perian's Place, SAFPAW's transitional recovery home for women and foster animals as they shift from homelessness to independent living. While in residence, the women contribute to running the household. They take care of all of the day-to-day chores and learn basic skills for financial responsibility, conflict resolution, and health care.

I asked Laurie if she has suffered physically from the manual labor she's done over so many years. "No way," she said, "I'm better off because of my time in the field. I don't give a flip what society thinks I should look like. I can pick up a sixty-pound, stray pit bull and put him in my car, no problem."

Though not Catholic, Laurie told me that one of her greatest inspirations is Mother Teresa. "She had a small stature, but she did things a person her size and age 'shouldn't' be able to do—and she did them because she didn't see an excuse. She didn't say, 'I'm short, I'm old,' you know? She wasn't going to let anything stop her. Her attitude was that if everyone took care of those around them, her work wouldn't have been necessary.

"The problem is that we have a failure to connect with the people in our own backyards. I'd rather be at a homeless camp than a cocktail party. When I went down to tent city for the first time, I married my two true loves, which are animals and working with people who never had what I had growing up. I was adopted. If my birth mother had kept me, I could very well have ended up just like them. Her husband left her, and she didn't have an education. She had no way of supporting me. There's no difference between the people in the camps and me, you know? It's just luck, so I help where I can."

Laurie Green is beauty, and her example is an inspiration to exercise in productive, dynamic ways.

Every time we move, we improve the ways we function, and every time we connect with people "in our own backyards," we nurture not only them, but ourselves. Laurie is "exercising" in ways that haven't occurred to most of us, and her body is holding up better than most because she's done the work to keep herself strong, without even noticing that was what she was doing.

Exercise, as we know it, is a bizarre construct. If you love weight lifting or running, that's great. It's a gift. But *exercise* can also mean gardening, swimming, yoga, tai chi, taekwondo, biking, climbing, softball, canoeing, cleaning your apartment, stacking boxes at a food pantry, hiking, rock climbing, horseback riding, bathing animals at a rescue, helping a friend move, distributing pamphlets, registering people to vote, gathering wildflowers, or the most magical (and totally free) exercise of all—walking.

If you specifically want to gain strength, yes, there might be some squats in your future, but the only reason to do them is because you like how they make you feel. If you despise them or if you're doing them the wrong way and putting your health in jeopardy, there are a bajillion other ways to get healthier and stronger.

TOO MUCH EXERCISE CAN BE JUST AS DAMAGING AS NOT ENOUGH

Cait Snow is a thirty-five-year-old professional triathlete from Massachusetts. She knows a lot about exercising for the right reasons and for the wrong ones. She competed in her first triathlon when she was twelve and has been hooked ever since. Cait has completed twenty-two full Ironman events and won two of them, and she has raced in the Ironman World Championships eight times, placing in the top ten four times.

She could definitely destroy me in a game of dodgeball.

But a few years ago, at the height of her career, she began to disconnect from the training. She was tired and hungry. She started feeling depleted rather than invigorated by the competition. "I remember being in Hawaii racing at the Ironman World Championship," she said, "some of the last rides I was doing before race day, I would ride by the airport thinking, 'Okay, one more week and you can get on a plane and go back home and be away from this pressure and eat whatever you want,' instead of thinking how awesome it was that I got to compete in the Championship against the best athletes in the world in one of the most beautiful places in the world. That should have been something I was pumped about, but all I could think about was my body composition—I couldn't keep going full-throttle to make sure everybody was happy or impressed."

Professional triathletes don't make a salary. They win prize money if they win a race and can get sponsorships; but it's a constant pursuit to stay at the top of their game to attract sponsors and qualify for more races. Round and round they go, always looking to the next event.

Cait's goal was to get down to 12 percent body fat for race days. She tracked everything she ate for years in extensive Excel documents. She thought that if she didn't track every workout and every morsel of food, she would get to the starting line "fat" and be unable to perform.

When I spoke with her, she hadn't had her period in seven years. Her doctor had just detected early signs of osteoporosis and prescribed a new estrogen treatment to get her period going. The pressure drove her to binge at night, and she woke up in the mornings guilty and ashamed.

She told me, "People look at athletes and think they are specimens of ultimate health, but the folks on the covers of magazines or on the podium aren't necessarily in great health. I see it especially in female athletes in running and triathlon; they don't fuel their workouts because it's an easy way to lose weight, but they also start to lose muscle. Their bodies start to break down, and they get injured—injuries that are not normal, like a stress fracture in the pelvis or something. That bone should be so freaking dense that you'd have to fall from a high height to fracture it. The competition gets so intense."

More isn't always better. There is such a thing as enough, and there is such a thing as a healthy body weight. There doesn't always have to be another pound to lose, and we don't have to be consumed by an eternal battle with our appetites.

Cait remembers watching video footage of an Ironman race she won early in her career. Friends watching with her ripped on the woman who came in third. They ridiculed her, saying "imagine how much better she would be if she just lost a little weight." The woman they spoke of is a champion competitor. She has completed sixty Ironman triathlons. I have seen the photos of that race, and it boggles the mind that anyone had anything to say other than *Killer finish!*

According to Cait, "In this field, if your body jiggles at all, you are judged. I'm constantly wondering, 'What are people thinking? Do they think I'm fat?' I don't want to admit I'm thinking that way, but I am."

Cait's story kills me. Not just because of the damage she was doing to her body in the name of fitness, but because her story is typical. She's not alone. I can't speak to the Ironman community she knows so well. That isn't my world, but I can speak to the experience of regular people who are just trying to get in shape. So many of us are seeking un-jiggly perfection, but our bodies will never fit the bill. We are mammals, and we require fat to function optimally. What Cait has been able to accomplish as an athlete is extraordinary, but she wasn't able to appreciate the best of it because her whole life became a game of *harder, faster, THINNER!* Exercise became an obsession and an obligation, and she lost contact with the purpose of it all, good health.

I hear stories like hers all the time from regular people who aren't athletes, who sign up for boot camp out of the blue or decide to work out twice a day, five times a week, after being sedentary for years. Most of the time, these people get injured, or at least burned out, long before any of their goals are reached. And the predictable cycle of guilt and frustration ensues before they call it a fail and give up entirely.

Cait pushed her body until it started breaking down, but now, finally, she is learning to listen to what it's trying to tell her. She stepped away from triathlons this year. Instead, she'll compete in seventeen smaller races as part of an organization called More Than Sport that raises money for clean water, shelter, food, medicine, and education.[3]

"A big part of it is to raise money," she said, "but another big part is to take the pressure off. The stress I'm putting myself under is becoming physically unhealthy. I need to get in touch with my intuition again. You get to a point where you kind of block it out. I'm used to pushing myself to beyond fatigue, and now I'm learning to listen again. I lost sight of the joy and fun and excitement at being able to do these things with my body. Now, whenever I go for a run or a hike or a bike ride or whatever, I try to remember, 'Wow, Cait, isn't this amazing that you're able to do this? You don't have to push any harder than you're pushing. You're fine. You don't have to go any faster. Look at what you're doing with your body. It's awesome.'"

GIVE YOUR BODY CREDIT WHERE CREDIT IS DUE

It's sobering to realize that even some of the most fit among us beat themselves up for not being good enough or slim enough. I see it in my clients, too. "Thin" people aren't necessarily any more at peace with their bodies than heavier ones. We're all in this mess together, no matter our weight.

In an international study commissioned by Dove in 2016, researchers interviewed 10,500 women in thirteen countries to understand how they viewed their bodies. The study "reveals the impact low body-esteem has on a woman's ability to realize her potential, with huge percentages of women (85%) and girls (79%) saying they opt out of important life activities—such as trying out for a team or club and engaging with family or loved ones—when they don't feel good about the way they look. Additionally, 7 in 10 girls with low body-esteem say they won't be assertive in their opinion or stick to their decision if they aren't happy with the way they look."[4]

Low self-esteem and bad body image impact every sphere of life, and if we aren't happy with the way we look *no matter how we look*, it would seem we're engaged in a losing battle. The negative repercussions will spread through our education and earning potential as well as our health. So forget it. Turn your attention to what your body can *do*, regardless how you think it looks. The image you hold in your head is probably flawed anyway. Focusing on the capabilities you do have will make you a whole lot stronger in the long run than nitpicking all the ways you do not resemble Lupita Nyong'o.

Make a list of what is working for you and pay homage to one or more of those body parts. Every. Day.

In case you hadn't noticed, not everyone can stand up and cheer at a baseball game or a Broadway musical. That requires smooth joints, a strong back, powerful legs, a brain to comprehend what is happening, and enthusiasm for a helluva slider or a helluva song. Take a moment every day to notice what *doesn't* hurt in your body. It is a huge gift *not* to be suffering with stomach or muscular issues. If you haven't ever experienced debilitating or persistent pain, you are likely a shining example of what old folks mean when they say, "Youth is wasted on the young." A healthy, functional body is an extraordinary asset. Lavish all kinds of love on what you've got, every day, before you waste time berating yourself for what you don't have.

If there are old aches and pains you don't have any more, remember what they felt like and compare that to how you feel now. If there are new aches and pains you didn't used to have, spend some time appreciating and reinforcing the parts of your body that feel good, while looking for active ways to heal or manage your discomfort.

While you're at it, have a look back at old photos from your teenage years to check out how young and vital you were when you first started ripping your appearance to shreds, and consider for a minute that your perspective might be as misguided now as it was back then.

Make a list of your favorite activities and the physical capabilities required to accomplish them.

If you are an amateur photographer, you lift your arms and hold them steady. You look at a shot with clear eyes and crouch down to get just the right angle.

If you love to bike, your legs propel you up steep hills and your lungs respond with rhythmic, continuous breath. If you have to hop off the bike and push it up the hill, the same legs and lungs are getting the job done, just in a different way.

If you cook, you're on your feet, bending and reaching and stirring all day. You traipse all over town looking for the right ingredients and spend hours pulling it all together so you can feed yourself and/or the people you love.

Give your body the respect it deserves. Feel free to indulge in an ongoing diatribe in your mind, your own private celebration of all the awesome ways your body shows up for you every day. There are a million muscles and bones and nerves in your body making things happen. You won't run out of helpful body parts to be thankful for any time soon.

Last, make a list of ways to push yourself. Make physical challenges integral to your confidence and self-care.

If you can't reach your toes in a forward fold, visit that position for sixty seconds every night before bed and watch what happens over weeks and months.

If you want to run a 10K but can only run for three minutes before gasping for air, run for three and walk for three and repeat until you're ready to run for four and walk for two.

If you're totally out of shape and haven't moved in years, just start walking. Every day. Fifteen minutes. Or sign up for a beginner's yoga class. Or tai chi. Or get a membership at one of those giant trampoline places and jump around a couple times a week.

And while you're doing any or all of those things, try to remember what you loved to do as a kid. If you used to love horses but are uncomfortable getting on one now, volunteer at stables that bring city kids and horses together for therapy. Find some variation of what you love and get yourself moving. The point is to get off your tush by doing something that feeds your heart and soul. If you can do that, you win.

NO SUCH THING AS PERFECT

Making the shift to appreciating your body rather than picking it apart is easier said than done, but it helps to notice that you're not alone in this predicament. And you can get high on an internal power trip when you realize that the choice of whether to vilify your body or not is *100 percent up to you*. You don't have to do it anymore if you don't want to.

You know who else isn't perfectly un-jiggly? Everyone. Literally everyone. Even people we think of as physically flawless catch hell for their bodies, no matter how fit they are. The world is full of people with opinions about how women's bodies are supposed to look, but when it comes down to it, the only opinions that matter are our own.

Lady Gaga can show us the way. She sets a stellar example for how not to give a damn. She puts her body and her creativity in the bull's-eye for millions of internet trolls who try to tear her down—and she keeps right on going.

When she performed at the Super Bowl in 2016, her performance was fierce, and I was aghast the next day to discover that the internet exploded with insults about her body. I saw a talented, fit, athletic, and very slim woman performing dance moves it would take me years to master while belting out chart-topping hits that would have me gasping for air—but a terrifyingly large portion of the population saw a fat stomach. It's called flesh, people. It's called health.

Twelve percent body fat and washboard abs are not normal, nor are they necessarily healthy. I doubt it occurred to Gaga to question her outfit before that performance, and we know she didn't second-guess it afterward because she sent a message to her "Little Monsters" via Instagram. "I heard my body is a topic of conversation so I wanted to say, I'm proud of my body and you should be proud of yours, too. . . . Be you, and be relentlessly you. That's the stuff of champions."

A few months later, she revealed that she suffers severe pain from fibromyalgia, making her passion and agility onstage all the more remarkable. What Gaga does with her body in performance is not only athletically impressive, it is a pure expression of her joy, perseverance, and, sometimes, outrage.

THE BEST EXERCISE IS ONE YOU CAN LOVE

The exercise that makes the most sense for you is whatever kind lights you up. If you haven't figured out what that is yet, keep trying new things until you find it, and always remember it doesn't have to require grueling hours on a treadmill. It can also change over time. The purpose of working out is *to rejuvenate you*, not to manage or control your body. Exercise can be dancing or dog walking, rock climbing or karate, yoga or competitive karaoke. When we let go of what we "should" be doing, we can figure out what we actually *like* doing—and that's the key to keeping ourselves agile and quick.

One of the best examples I know of a woman who has found an unusual and fantastic form of exercise to love is Ginger. Ginger grew up as part of a baseball family, Cubs fans from Illinois. She tried to play in a Little League when she was seven, but the coach and other players excluded her every time the kids paired off to practice throwing and catching. She was forced out after half a season, so at eight, she joined a softball team instead. She says she wasn't very good at first, but the following year she was named Most Improved Player and became Most Valuable Player for three years running after that. She played in various softball leagues from high school through her thirties, but in her forties, she found her center of gravity in vintage base ball.

According to the Vintage Base Ball Association's website, vintage base ball (two words, not one) promotes "living history by bringing the 19th century to life through base ball events that use the rules, equipment, costumes and culture of the 1860s. Our goal is to exemplify, to youth and adults alike, the values that are lacking in modern-day athletic programs, and encourage a sense of belonging regardless of race, gender, religious conviction or physical ability."[5]

There are twelve teams in her league, with only five women out of 180 "ballists." They play bare-handed. Gloves and other protective gear weren't introduced until later. On game day, participants go out to an empty field to measure and chalk the baselines. They set up a handmade wooden and chicken-wire backstop with benches and period-style tents for the teams to sit under. Fans bring lawn chairs and picnics, and a band plays period music during the breaks to set the mood. "Setting up the game is a fantastic experience," she says.

Ginger walks, jogs, and has recently started lifting weights during the off-season to improve her performance on game days, but she says, "Playing two or three hours of base ball doesn't seem like exercise to me at all. It's my happy place. It reminds me of the old adage, 'If you do something you love, you'll never work a day in your life.' Exercise is a fringe benefit of playing ball. I do the other stuff to make the base ball easier."

When she's not on the field, Ginger is the adult programs director at her local library. She plans events with specialists in a wide variety of fields, and she loves the job. Some of her favorites have included a volunteer from the Elephant Sanctuary; a Beatles scholar ("music, not bugs"); and various health-related events. In addition to bringing civility back to sports and enriching the cultural experience of her community, she is ushering her two kids through middle school.

Ginger has found her "thing" and thrills at the thought of donning her vintage uniform before each game. "It is invigorating to play. My hands sometimes bruise, but less as I have gotten used to different ways to catch. I hold myself to pretty high standards. We are out there to have fun, but I also want to perform well. Even on days that we don't win, it's always a joy to have played. It's my favorite way to spend a day."

EAT FOR YOUR BODY. EXERCISE FOR YOUR MIND.

Exercise is for boosting your mood. It is for taking you out of your head and into your body. Yes, it will improve your body composition and all of the delicate systems that keep you alive, but the end result of that improvement is that you'll feel better, feel sharper, and have more energy to devote to your work, to your family and friends, and to changing whatever injustice in the world you simply can't tolerate any longer.

I lift moderate weights a couple of times a week because *I like it*. It makes me feel strong. I go to yoga once a week because it keeps me sane and limber. I walk every day because I'm tense and sluggish if I don't and because I get my best ideas while my heart is pumping extra blood to my brain. Those are my things. Even though I'm a trainer, I don't feel the need to run a single mile. Running doesn't feel useful for my body, except in rare moments when it feels like breaking free, and when those moments arrive, I listen.

Your body is unique. The ways you respond to different kinds of exercise are unique. As long as you're trying to squeeze yourself into someone else's definition of fit, you're making a mess of your fitness plans.

It has to be fun, and you have to find your own way to do what works for you. You need comfortable activities you can do with your eyes closed *and others that challenge you.*

Progress lives in the edges around your comfort zones. Your body can do more than you think it can. Give it a chance to try. Creep around just beyond your boundaries to see what else you might like to do. Moving in your body will allow you to move in your mind, and it will enable you to keep moving forward in your life as well. Comfort is important. We need places we can retreat to, where we can rest, but if we live there all the time, we are missing out on everything else—whatever that might be. If we stop moving, our muscles atrophy, our joints stiffen, and our minds corrode.

When I find myself staring at the computer, fruitlessly trying to force my creative mind to work, I have learned to step away and take my dog for a walk down a street I've never been down before. I see cats and yard art. I see flowers and trees. I see neighbors wheeling up wheelchair ramps, kids skateboarding, and elderly couples sitting on porch swings. I get a shot of vitamin D without breaking the skin. And when I come back home, I have something new on my mind, something worth exploring.

When that doesn't work, I go for the coup de grâce, the death-blow to my stagnant creativity, a life-changing exercise I call *kvetching and stretching*. The only ingredients required to jump-start your body and brain are a friend and a floor. Put down the computer. Step away from the TV and the treadmill. Stretch. Talk and laugh about shit that matters and shit that doesn't matter with someone who gives a damn while you try to get a tiny bit closer to touching your toes and a little bit looser in your hips.

I promise you'll come away with a brand-new idea about something you never thought of before. And your back will hurt a lot less, too.

Fill in the Blank

This exercise sucks and I am not going to do it any more: _____
_____.

An unconventional kind of exercise I'd like to try is _____
_____.

I'm going to schedule it for _____

_____ .

Some ways I can move more that aren't technically *exercise* are

_____

_____ .

I am going to stretch every day for five minutes before/after I

_____ .

When I'm trying to work on _____

but can't think straight, I will _____

_____ to get my body and brain moving.

By moving, we are
waking our bodies up, not
making them surrender.

CHAPTER 6

Food as Medicine

Sorry to say it, but we're even more messed up about food than we are about exercise.

My own noxious relationship with food began in the seventh grade. My best friend and I would run to the cafeteria before it filled up with our classmates, pile our lunch trays high with spaghetti, garlic bread, and brownies, and sneak down to the bowels of the auditorium to eat. We hunched over our lunches, talking about how we hoped the boys didn't see what was on our plates as we scurried past them on the way out. I ate Pop Tarts for breakfast and heaping spoonfuls of cookie dough after dinner—sugar to start the day and sugar to finish.

In high school, I had "dinner" at my boyfriends' houses more times than I can count, eating only a few pieces of lettuce and claiming not to be hungry, and wrote letters to the editors of teen magazines, wondering about the calorie count of toothpaste and cough syrup.

When I went to college, a group of aspiring ballet dancers shared with me the wonders of laxatives and diuretics. I began hiding boxes of cookies from roommates at the back of my closet. Lunchtime in the cafeteria became a side salad with fat-free dressing, *or* an apple, *or* a bowl of Cap'n Crunch. I knew I was getting somewhere when upon exiting the lunch room an upperclassman said, "Hey, if your ass gets any smaller, I'm going to have to get to know you better."

Success.

I was a regular encyclopedia of warped ways to handle food: Ten animal crackers equal one serving. Club soda is super filling in combination with a six-pack of yeast rolls. If you want to get buzzed, marijuana is better than beer because it doesn't have any calories, but watch out for the munchies. Sleeping with guys helps you avoid late night binges because, of course, you would never eat in front of them—unless you get lucky and can sneak a snack out of the closet while they're passed out. It's okay to eat an extra-large order of French fries (or two) if you order at the drive-through window and eat in the parking lot next door, preferably facing a tall concrete wall with the sun visor pulled down. Don't forget the ketchup or you'll have to take the walk of shame into the restaurant with your hoodie up.

The situation caught up with me in New York City after graduation. Burritoville, Jackson Hole Diner, and Krispy Kreme became my very best friends. Isolation became far more comfortable than companionship, and by twenty-two, I was binging and purging several times a day.

Don't panic. I don't have much to say about puking, except that it's a symptom of the problem we've been discussing all along: We misunderstand beauty, placing it on the outside, skinny and spackled. We have fleshy bodies with stubborn "imperfections." To remedy that situation, we turn food into forbidden fruit, and all we want from then on out is one enormous, coma-inducing bite after another. We get so distracted by what to eat and what not to eat that we lose track of who we are and what we're passionate about. And decades pass.

FINDING YOUR BALANCE

A client recently asked me if it's possible to be "in balance" with regard to her relationship with food, or if the goal she should be shooting for is to learn how to be okay with being out of balance. What she meant was: *Is it possible for mealtime to be about genuine hunger and satisfaction, instead of discipline and shame? Or is the best case scenario that I stop being so freaked out by discipline and shame, and let them exist innocuously alongside my lasagna?* A few years ago, I would have told her that being at peace with being out of balance is the ultimate goal, but over time, I have learned that balance—eating free of guilt and anxiety—is absolutely possible.

Being okay with being out of balance is the *first* goal (and a crucial one), but there is such a thing as being in balance, in love with food, and in love with your body. I've been on all sides of this equation. I have hated food, made peace with being out of sync with it, and finally found joy in it. These days, I eat healthy *and* unhealthy foods in the right proportions to satisfy my grown-up self and my little-kid-with-a-popsicle-under-the-porch self. It keeps me content and flexible. I have abandoned the concept of physical or dietary perfection in exchange for an evolving sense of which foods feel right in my body and which foods feel wrong. This requires listening, but it also requires stumbling, falling, thirsting, craving, recovering, savoring, and continuing on.

I hate to cook. I wish I liked it, but I don't. I don't have the attention span for it. I don't make the time and truthfully don't have much desire to try. I'd be useless without pre-made sauces that come in a jar and pre-mixed spices that come in a tin. I do love vegetables, which helps a lot with striking a balance, but I have a hard time finding inspiration in the kitchen. My husband fires up the grill a couple of times a year, and I make some sort of boxed, organic risotto and oven-roasted veggie to fill out the meal. We get by, but cooking is definitely not an art form at my house. If you love to cook, bonus points, but if you don't, you won't get any flak from me.

You are what you eat, which makes me a plate of Indian take-out with a broccoli floret for a head and blocks of dark chocolate for feet, and that sounds perfect to me. It's a celebration of everything I love and the freedom I've found to enjoy it—so distant from the hatred I had for food and my body for most of my life.

• • •

When I bring up diet with my clients, I usually get a knee-jerk response that they can't change it. *Tried. Failed. Too hard. Can't stick with it. Don't cook. Can't find time. Cravings too strong. Willpower too weak.* All of these things have been true for them in the past. They feel as if these are immutable truths, hard facts, but the reason their attempts to change their diets have failed is because they were trying to apply diet plans like a doctor would prescribe antibiotics. *Take this dose. Follow this plan, and you'll be fixed.*

But it's not that simple. Any prescribed list of what you can and cannot eat—based not on allergies or nutritional requirements, but on a food's "fat burning capacity" or its potential to send you into ketosis—separates you from hearing what your body is trying to tell you and giving it what it needs.

We need food. We can't quit it.

You have to eat, and the only "fix"—the only method that will work to establish a balanced relationship with food—is to become aware of how different foods interact with your physical and emotional well-being. And then do what works FOR YOU. Once you can perceive *for yourself* which choices don't sit well with your body and mind, you can make the decision not to eat those things because of the price you pay, not because of how they might make you look or because you're "not supposed to" eat them.

Hard and fast rules don't work for most of us, especially when they are determined by someone other than us, as individuals. How your body reacts to different food changes over time, too. The only approach that will serve you for the rest of your life is to understand:

- **Intellectually** that food is the essential fuel that keeps you alive and alert. It provides the building

blocks for your basic survival and your master plan
for world domination.

- And **viscerally** the difference between how you feel
when you feed yourself fatty, sugary, unwieldy food
and when you feed yourself satisfying, life-giving
food.

Don't forget, I'm the one who buys all the pre-cut ingredients and
pre-made sauces. I'm not talking about extreme "clean eating" where
you have to make everything from scratch from the gardens and hens
in your own backyard. I'm talking about knowing that the ingredients in your food still resemble the substances they were when they
arrived on planet Earth. Of course, you can keep eating delicious and
easy things out of boxes, as long as they contain ingredients that exist
in nature. The fresher the better, but who the hell has time to grow,
pick, wash, chop, assemble, cook, and eat totally fresh every single
day?? Not me. That's for sure.

The food we eat has an enormous impact on our bodies and minds.
Every scrap of good juju you can put into your body makes a difference. Understanding what you're choosing to eat and why is important, but dissecting your diet all the time can feel like trying to climb
a limestone cliff coated in Astroglide. Slip and fall.

What's most important is quieting some of the noise around the
food landscape.

When you get to thinking about this in the context of your own
body, you only really need to answer one question: Does it make you
feel better or worse when you eat it?

Listen to that.

FOOD CAN BE HEALING

Food has the capacity to heal us physically and psychologically, and
we don't have to compete for *Top Chef* to win the grand prize: a healthy

body and an easy relationship with food. You can change the way you feel by changing what you put in your body.

Severe food allergies can be dangerous and even life-threatening, and mild allergies or sensitivities can make you feel legit lousy. Even if you don't have allergies, you probably know all too well which foods slow you down and which ones boost your energy. A friend of mine swears he can take on the world after eating a plateful of sashimi but caffeine sends him into a tailspin of grumpy, aggressive behavior.

According to Dr. Forbes, MD, board certified integrative holistic physician, and former president of the American Holistic Medical Association, the vast majority of us can improve our chronic conditions and reduce our suffering simply by adjusting our diets. It's a tool we ignore at our own peril.

"We, as a medical culture, don't have any recognition of how many drugs we are throwing at food problems, mainly in the form of stomach, anxiety, depression, and sinus medications." He told me that most of his patients, after making a few straightforward dietary changes, "come back in and tell me some variation of, 'I feel so much better. I can't believe food was doing this to me.'"

The way he treats these complaints might vary from person to person, but the goal is to help his patients discover which foods reduce their symptoms and allow their bodies to thrive. He frequently approaches his patients' problems by clearing the deck of food triggers that might be causing difficulty and building those foods back in to see what causes symptoms or discomfort and what doesn't. "I'm trying to get them to tune in to listening and paying attention to how they feel," he says.

• • •

So how can each of us find symptoms that might be associated with food and figure out which parts of our diets are causing them? The answer to that question is both totally complicated and very simple. There is no one-size-fits-all solution. There is also no quick-fix method to find out what is causing indigestion or bloating. Allergy testing can be useful if you think you're sensitive to specific foods, but both skin prick and blood tests can yield false positives.

Again, what matters is what feels right. If you think cutting out one or several kinds of food might make you feel better, experimenting can certainly be beneficial—but don't make yourself crazy trying to adhere to rules that make you miserable or that you have no intention of following.

In a perfect world, eating should provide some combination of sustenance and celebration. So as you look for ways to feed yourself better, remember that the point is to invigorate your body. That's all. Dig around in your diet and root out some changes, but don't get lost in the weeds.

When we make food the enemy, we always lose.

WHERE TO START

The easiest way to figure out if a particular type of food is making you feel terrible is to do a gut check, literally, and try eliminating one food at a time to see if it helps with any symptoms over the course of two or three weeks. ONE food at a time. To do this, try keeping a journal for a few weeks *before* you make any change, to document when symptoms arise (including mood and sleep issues) and what foods might have triggered them—usually within the last twenty-four hours, but it can take longer. For example, the next time you're sluggish in the middle of the day or your stomach is churning all morning, think through things like this:

Did you eat a bucket of pasta last night and a bunch of white bread? Feeling sluggish and depressed today by any chance?

Did you eat a salad you thought was awesome and healthy for lunch but an hour later you're doubled over on the toilet? Was there cheese in that salad? Does the same thing happen when you have pizza? You may have a dairy problem. Maybe, maybe not, but it's worth experimenting to find out.

If you can find a likely cause and effect, you can cut out the suspected food and keep the journal going to see if there are any changes. After several weeks, if you like the way you feel, stick with it. If it hasn't made a difference, that food may be completely fine for you. Let it go, and move on.

This method isn't as sweeping as a full elimination diet where you cut out all of the possible triggers at once, but it's a lot more manageable and a good way to start if you think you have a food sensitivity. The key is to be vigilant about the change (*just that one*) and stick with it long enough to see results or lack thereof.

Most of us know when something isn't treating our bodies right. We get queasy every time we have ice cream, bread, or beer. We feel heavy and bloated or foggy and exhausted—but we really, *really* don't want to consider that our favorite food might be the culprit. So we take lactose pills/acid reducers/energy drinks and keep on with the same old habits until the problem gets so bad that we can't stand it anymore, at which point we call the doc for prescription pills. Non-digestive symptoms like joint pain, headaches, depression, eczema, and nagging cough or nasal congestion can be even harder to identify because they might be food-related or they might be brought on by a smear of environmental, viral, bacterial, stress-induced, genetic, or other causes.

Sorting through all of that is a steep climb, so a lot of us resign ourselves to feeling vaguely miserable when something as simple as eating *more* of a healthy group of foods might make us feel so much better. It's disconcerting to try a new routine, especially around something like food, which is so tied to our emotional lives. Changing anything about the way you eat always feels unsteady at first, but if you're making one change at a time—and your stomach and mind are benefiting from it—you can breathe and sleep and wake up ready for whatever is on the agenda: small decisions about what to eat or bigger ones about whether to brush up your resume or move to the Netherlands.

If you can heal your body by changing your diet, you're not only avoiding the hassle and side effects of taking drugs to Band-Aid over recurring problems, you're also saving money. Healthy food is much cheaper than drugs and hospitals and doctors. And when you do make a dietary change stick—and it increases your energy or helps you lose a few pounds—you see how profound the effect of food is on your body and get inspired to keep going, feeding yourself as often as possible with food that heals.

CLEARING OUT

One of the best parts of what I get to do for a living is watch my clients, after months of preparation, launch into new versions of themselves, awakening lifeblood they never knew they had. It's even better when I'm not optimistic about their odds, and they totally prove me wrong. A client named Rosa taught me never to make assumptions about what people are capable of when they get a taste of feeling better.

Rosa reached out to me about two years ago via email, saying "I'm forty-three years old, five foot seven inches, and currently weigh 250 lbs. My weight has been a battle all my life. I know what I should be doing. I just can't seem to put it all together. After neglecting myself for years, I have a huge challenge ahead of me. I know this won't be easy, but I am ready to work. My biggest concern is finding someone who is also able to provide some insight with the mental challenge I know this will be."

Rosa described being hounded with obsessive thoughts and overwhelming anxiety about causing pain or disappointment to the people she cares about most. She also had a whole bunch of stomach, skin, and sinus issues that were getting worse over the course of many years. When we started working together, she came into our sessions distracted and evasive. She complained a lot about work and feeling lethargic, and deflected my suggestions about making incremental dietary changes. She drank numerous diet sodas every day and chose unhealthy options at her work cafeteria. She also frequently made fast-food pit stops on the way to and from work.

Her diet was off the table at the beginning, but she *was* interested in addressing her stiff muscles and aching joints. So, in addition to our workouts once a week, she started pursuing other ways to support her body, by seeing a massage therapist and chiropractor regularly.

Rosa progressed this way for about a year but didn't say much during our workouts about her relationship with food or her body. I didn't press her, not verbally anyway, but over time, I did begin to push her harder in our sessions. She grew stronger and more capable of responding to new exercises than before. We were able to make real progress with her strength and endurance, but her weight continued to rise.

Finally, after several rounds of prescription steroids for a chest cold she couldn't kick, continual digestive issues, raging plantar fasciitis, and losing the natural curl in her hair, she came in one morning and said, "Something is wrong with me. Something is really wrong. I know it sounds weird, but losing my curls is the last straw. I need to do something."

She went to see Dr. Forbes and decided to go on a full elimination diet to try to figure out what could be triggering her issues, especially her digestive problems. I was skeptical at best, but she was determined to cut grains, soy, corn, dairy, sugar, and alcohol out of her diet completely and headed to the health food store the following weekend with an unfamiliar shopping list in hand.

She said the first week "Sucked. There's no way around it." It was tough, but after a couple of days, she noticed that her mind was clearer than it had been in years—and that was a perk she never anticipated. Curiosity about whether the clarity would remain got her through to week two, when she began to notice other ailments improving system-wide. The cravings began to dissipate. She was sleeping better. Her energy shot up, and her mind was less burdened with each passing day.

By the end of week three, Rosa told me, "I wake up every day and feel better than the day before. My joints don't hurt. Movement feels better. My skin tone and texture are improved. No more hives or rashes. I'm waking up with energy instead of dull headaches and brain fog. Concentration is better. Sinuses are clear for the first time I can remember. My IBS issues are starting to get better. There's no more swelling in my feet and legs, and I'm finally losing weight."

As she continued over the course of many months, she made adjustments and added several of the foods back in, purposefully and one at a time. But the most important resource she gained was an intuitive sense of her body and its needs.

Changing her diet freed her from a multitude of ailments, and, as of this writing, Rosa has lost thirty pounds. "I'm sticking with it for now," she says. "I just really want to know how much better I can feel. There are days when I struggle, but I'm successful in figuring out ways to manage it. I'm staying focused on the benefits I'm seeing."

The benefits. The symptoms she was enduring before she made the changes were enough to motivate her through that first week, but then *the benefits* took over and far outweighed the effort it took to keep going. Rosa felt great—a little conflicted and weird (because change is weird) but, overall, so much better.

I was astonished that she stuck with it and continued sorting through which changes were useful and which could go by the wayside. Diets like Rosa's can backfire, causing people to slingshot back to their old demons if they're focused on what they can't have. But Rosa was focused on what she *could* have: a body that feels better.

The biggest reason her new eating patterns stuck is because she committed fully to the cardinal rule about any dietary change: **She stayed full.** She didn't starve herself. Unable to eat the food she used to eat, she branched out, trying new recipes and figuring out how to get enough fiber and protein to stay satisfied. Achieving true "balance" will take a while longer, but she is well on her way.

For reasons known only to Rosa, she was ready to scrap her old way of eating and try something entirely new. She cleared the deck, and it worked for her. It allowed her to tune in to how an unhealthy diet was destroying her well-being and a healthier one could improve it, far beyond weight loss. And the changes she made have opened up a whole other world for her. She can work with greater focus now and love with greater openness. She has figured out how to stop contributing to her own destruction and start contributing to her strengths.

THE BASICS

Food is the stuff of life. If we feed ourselves trash, we feel like trash. If we eat heavy, we feel heavy.

When it comes to our energy levels, mental sharpness, and, of course, our waistlines, food is paramount.

Personally, I have never been successful with anything even approaching the path that Rosa took. Even now, if I tried to do something like that, I would panic and start hording sweets in the dark again. It wouldn't be healthy for me psychologically. But I *have* been successful permanently weaning myself off foods that make me feel gross, and those are huge wins. Over many years, responding to what my body tells me about specific foods has changed what my diet looks like and what my body feels like:

If I eat even a small hit of sugar after lunch, I'm always dragging ass by 3 p.m.

If I eat any amount of chocolate after 8 p.m., there is no chance that I will be able to fall asleep before midnight.

If I eat a piece of fruit or a handful of nuts midafternoon, I'm always more satisfied after dinner and much less likely to crave empty snacks before bed.

And if I don't eat probiotic yogurt and flaxseed granola for breakfast (or take a probiotic supplement if I'm on the road), I will definitely be constipated and irritable all day. I'm sure any day now I'll be eating prunes in a rocking chair. Don't care. Whatever makes my body function better works for me.

I don't eat meat or poultry because they freak me out, but I do eat fish begrudgingly because it makes me feel better. I use unsweetened almond milk for my morning tea (and everything else I might use milk for), but I still eat organic cheese and yogurt. I don't stick to vegan or paleo or Mediterranean. The only "diet" these parameters fit into is my own—and none of this information about my diet should have any relevance to yours.

Do what works for you, but whatever you do, don't let anybody sell you on a bunch of expensive powders and pills that are supposed to "fix" you. A few supplements can be helpful to add to your diet if you're addressing a particular issue and if the benefits and the brand are well-established. The probiotic supplement I take is an example of one that works for me, but for the most part, real food does the trick.

I don't recommend specific supplements unless I'm one-on-one with a client, but it's worth checking with your doctor for routine screening of your vitamin D and B12 levels to make sure they're normal. A multivitamin can also be a good idea if you think you're not getting a wide enough variety of foods, but you don't need to bury yourself in nutritional concoctions or spend a bunch of money on supplements to be healthy.

Food has the capacity to hurt or heal. We hold enormous power in our hands every time we lift a bite of food into our mouths.

You can make whatever rules you like about what you're supposed to eat and not supposed to eat, but the basics are pretty straightforward. How does the food make you feel? Does it make you feel lighter or heavier? Does it make you feel addicted or out of control?

If a food makes you feel bad, that choice might not be so helpful. Other options are available, and the changes don't have to be extreme.

- Fill up on the good stuff instead of worrying too much about quitting the bad.

- Satisfy your hunger with fruits and vegetables, unsalted nuts, lean protein, healthy fat, and high-fiber, whole grains.
- Fill at least half of your plate at every meal with vegetables. It doesn't matter if they are cooked or raw, frozen or fresh, just watch out for creamy, buttery sauces.
- Don't go hungry, and you'll be much less likely to stuff yourself. Think of hunger on a scale of 1–10 (with 1 being starving and 10 being stuffed), and shoot to stay in the 4–6 range. Search online for "hunger scale" for more specific descriptions of the different levels of hunger.
- Take heed when your body responds negatively or you have aversions to specific foods.
- If you have an inkling that something in your diet might be making you sick, try a couple of weeks without it and see what happens. It doesn't have to be forever, just try it out and see if you feel better.

The process of cleaning out the cobwebs can take a while. Give yourself time. If you make a healthy change (big or small) and follow through with it, you'll feel the difference in ways you might not have expected. Your body and brain will function better, and you might even leave indigestion, headaches, or a few pounds behind along the way. But to make any kind of lasting change, you need to *have faith in yourself* and your ability to try a new way. Give your body a chance to find its equilibrium, to be nurtured and satisfied. Diet doesn't have to be a big deal.

WHICH FOODS ARE THE OFFENDERS?

I can't answer that for you. I can't call out specific foods because most of them are totally harmless for most people. Personally, I have a severe wheat allergy. The last time a restaurant "accidentally" served me a regular pizza instead of a gluten-free one, I was alone in a hotel room in Colorado and nearly ended up in the hospital after forty-eight hours of violent vomiting, diarrhea, and an inability to keep down so much as a sip of water. The only thing that stopped it was a sublingual pill my doctor called in to a random pharmacy that helps cancer patients undergoing chemo survive the nausea. That pill was heaven-sent. Wheat gives me giant rashes, too, and makes me want to disappear for weeks after ingesting it.

Sorry. TMI.

My point is that wheat is a nightmare for me, but I would never, ever tell my clients to go gluten-free. Whole grains can be nurturing, filling, and a wonderful part of a healthy diet. Everyone's body is different. People have strong opinions about dairy, eggs, meat, corn, soy, wheat, and sugar. But the only opinion that matters is your body's. If your body doesn't handle a specific food well, if it makes you feel bad, no one should ever tell you to eat it unless a doctor is altering your diet for medical reasons—and even then you have the right to a second opinion.

If eating peanuts or shellfish sends you into anaphylactic shock, you have a clear message that cannot be ignored. If you have milder symptoms, food might be the cause, and it might not. But if your gut tells you that it is, finding the source is well worth the effort—and avoiding that source of misery isn't all that difficult once you experience life without it.

If you don't have physiological "symptoms" per se, but you're just generally in a constant state of food hangover, you may not have a sensitivity at all. You may just be eating too much creamy, salty, sugary, high-fat, or dense caloric food with no nutrients. If that's the case, simply increasing the amount of fruits, vegetables, whole grains, and lean proteins in your diet at every meal and in-between meals can be transformative. It sounds impossibly uncomplicated, but it's true.

SUGAR

One of the quickest ways to throw off your equilibrium is to toss a bunch of refined sugar at it. When we talk about diet, it's impossible to avoid questions about sugar. It's seductive, and it hides everywhere—in salad dressings, crackers, peanut butter, cereal, pasta sauce, "protein" bars, and, of course, juices and sodas. You can find it under many names, including cane sugar, cane crystals, corn syrup, high fructose corn syrup, corn sweetener, glucose, fructose, dextrose, maltose, and so on. Our brains respond to it with persistent, seemingly uncontrollable cravings, especially when it is artificially added to processed food.

Sugar is the villain we hate to love, but we go right on loving it anyway. In large amounts it's completely terrible for us, but it is also one of the true pleasures in life. So I'm not inclined to make grandiose statements about the universal horrors of dessert.

Over the years, I've tried at least 550 times to quit sugar cold turkey and have never been successful. The only way I ever found to cut back was by connecting it directly with a consequence that was really bothering me, like the afternoon fatigue and late-night insomnia I mentioned before. Headaches and bloating are also reliable companions when I've had too much sugar. And—every time—when I eat it, I want more, which I find highly annoying because it takes me out of the driver's seat.

When I made those connections and cut back, I saw immediate results in my sleep and energy, but, to get there, I had to pay attention over months (and years) to notice how it was stimulating me and how much better I felt when I ate less of it. Then the choices became infinitely easier and smaller portions were much more satisfying.

Of course, sugar causes weight gain, but you may have noticed that weight *loss* doesn't seem to be enough of a motivator to persuade you to eat less of it. That's because weight loss takes too long, and it's wrapped up with a bunch of social, emotional, and dietary issues that have nothing to do with sugar. To figure out how to cut back directly on sugar, you need more immediate feedback to motivate your choices.

The most devastating impact of too many sweets that I've seen in my clients' lives, and my own, is the effect on our energy.

Eating sugar artificially boosts your energy level before sending it plummeting. The crash causes lethargy and, often, some level of depression.[1] You can see this roller coaster ride in kids on Halloween night. Adults are better able to manage the effects, but the physiological impact is the same.

According to Richard Johnson, a nephrologist at the University of Colorado Denver who was quoted in a *National Geographic* article called "Sugar Love: A Not So Sweet Tale," "Americans are fat because they eat too much and exercise too little. But they eat too much and exercise too little because they're addicted to sugar, which not only makes them fatter but, after the initial sugar rush, also saps their energy, beaching them on the couch."[2]

We are sick and tired because we're eating junk. So we eat more junk to boost our energy. It feels good for a second before making us sicker and more tired. That fatigue makes it hard to accomplish pretty much anything, so we eat more junk to get motivated—and the vicious cycle ensues.

Before making ambitious plans to lose weight, you have to address *fatigue* by giving your body the building blocks that it needs to function and not clobbering it with sugar every five seconds. You need vitamins, minerals, heart-healthy fats, whole carbohydrates, protein, water, fiber, and sleep. When you're not so sick and tired, you make better decisions, and a syrupy-sweet dessert starts to feel more like a kettlebell in the belly than a treat.

• • •

So what about fruit? It's sugary, right? Is it okay to eat it? I am not a religious person, but I need to go a little Garden of Eden on you here.

Fruit is literally a symbol of paradise. It is the bounty of the Earth, and any diet that tells you to quit fruit can suck it as far as I'm concerned.

Fruit is nurturing, magnificent food. The sugar in fruit (fructose) is balanced with water and fiber. It's a wonderful source of nutrients, and cutting it out—unless it's for explicit medical reasons—makes no sense to me. Apples and bananas aren't making you fat. You couldn't eat enough of them to put on weight. You would get way too full way too fast. Sugar is troublesome when it is artificially added—not when it's built into a whole, natural, beautiful piece of fruit. Frozen grapes or a sliced up melon can make great substitutes for dessert after dinner.

So, yes, added sugar can be addictive. When you're used to eating a lot of it, you want more because it offers fast energy but never quite satisfies you. It stimulates the same parts of the brain that respond to highly addictive drugs like cocaine and heroin—as do other reward-based activities like gambling and shopping—but reducing or quitting sugar will not send you to the emergency room with cold sweats and vomiting like heroin will. Added sugar isn't good for us, but it's not the devil either. It's a potent force with sneaky, deleterious effects on our bodies and minds, but we are not powerless to change the ways we use it. You can absolutely cut back (without freaking out) if you do it in ways that keep you satisfied.

The best way to satisfy a craving for sweets is through—first of all, of course—FRUIT. Second, honey and molasses won't spike your blood sugar like refined, white sugar or corn syrup will, and they also contain actual nutrients that your body can use, such as amino acids, vitamins, and minerals. They can be used in some recipes, replacing refined sugar, too, and will give you sweet satisfaction without as much negative impact, especially in combination with healthier, more filling flours like whole wheat, almond, or oat. But keep in mind that when calories from sugar (of any kind) get absorbed by our small intestines, all calories are the same.

If you can't make it through the night without a processed sugar fix, you are being held prisoner. It's an addiction that prohibits you from making independent choices based on what is best for your body and peace of mind. As we know, processed sugar doesn't just cause lethargy and weight gain. It also contributes to diseases such as diabetes and heart disease. The cycle has to end somewhere—either in the hospital or the kitchen. I prefer the kitchen, though you might have to drag me there kicking and screaming.

There are ways to eat sweet and healthy at the same time. If you can't deal with sugar cravings anymore—if you're tired of feeling out of control and don't *want* to deal with them anymore—you can find healthier ways to get your needs met. If you stay full and satisfied, the cravings will start to retreat on their own.

FILLING UP

As we've established, I'm no expert in the kitchen, so I went to talk to Laura Lea Goldberg, a certified holistic chef and author of *The Laura Lea Balanced Cookbook: 120+ Every Day Recipes for the Healthy Home Cook*, about inventive ways to eat healthy without going to extremes.

When I walked into her kitchen, she asked if it was okay if she cooked while we talked. "I think more clearly that way," she said. I watched in awe as she pulled out a food processor and proceeded to make a grab-and-go snack she called Minty Fudge Brownie Bites in less than fifteen minutes with nothing but a few raw ingredients and a freezer.[3] The ingredients were walnuts, dates, cocoa powder, coconut oil, sea salt, and peppermint and vanilla extracts.

She made this treat like I might boil water: mindlessly and quickly. At first I thought she was a superhero, but then I realized that I could probably make that recipe just as well if I could figure out how to assemble my food processor.

"I almost wish we could get the word *cook* out of our lexicon," she said, "because cooking implies that it's something complicated, and it really doesn't have to be like that. I mean I don't know anybody who doesn't have the time to take a can of wild tuna or salmon and put it on a bed of greens with some nuts and cheese or whatever and make a salad. Or you can buy healthy wraps or tortillas. You can make lettuce cups. You can put chicken in a Crock-Pot and eat that throughout the week. Cooking really doesn't have to be that complicated. Just keep it simple." The mantra on the back of her book is "No diet. No dogma. Just good food."

I asked this shaman of holistic eating about her relationship with sweets. She said, "I have a sweet tooth. Some people do better abstaining completely, but that's not me. I like to have sweet things around. I'm a good natural moderator, but I think that's because I fill myself up, you know?"

Yeah, Laura Lea Superhero, I do know. When I've had my handful of nuts or an apple with almond butter midday, I'm a lot less likely to end up with my face in the fridge after dinner looking for sugar (or salt for that matter), not because I'm forcing myself to stay away, but because my body has what it needs.

We can eat all day long and still be starving at night if the food we're eating has been stripped of nutrients and rendered lifeless. We can eat thousands of empty calories and find ourselves aching for more because our basic nutritional needs haven't been met. Yes, we should probably cut down on sugar, but the way to do that is by eating more real food, not by sheer will and determination.

But here's the thing, there are many shades of gray when it comes to the choices you make about your food. It's not all or nothing. You don't have to make drastic changes to make a big difference in how you feel. And over time, as your brain catches up to the changes happening in your body, you'll stay fuller and eat fewer calories and, probably, eventually settle at a lower weight. Small changes matter.

You can eat almost any vegetable either sautéed on the stove top or roasted in the oven. You can toss them in nothing but a little olive oil, sea salt, and crushed red pepper. If you want to get ambitious, you can add other spices such as oregano or rosemary. If you make up a big batch of veggies every few days, you can add them to every meal or eat them straight out of the fridge. Believe me, cooking this way takes only enough skill not to burn yourself, and if you're eating those veggies along with whatever you were going to eat anyway, you've made a huge step toward better nutrition *and toward filling up.*

You can eat out or get takeout regularly, too. Doing this healthfully is all about two things:

1. **Making a slightly better decision.** Skip the egg roll or the cheese sauce. Get something with veggies in it. Get the brown instead of the white rice or the whole wheat instead of the white bread. Send the bread basket back. Order a side salad instead of fries with your burger.

2. **Portion size.** Presented with a huge portion? Eat half and save half for your next meal, and fill up on a healthy snack if you get hungry in the meantime. Or split your entrée with somebody. *It is possible to do this if know you have a snack coming,* but the snacks have to be grabbable: nuts, fruit, hummus and carrots, Greek yogurt, or a homemade flourless banana oat muffin. Half of an almond butter sandwich with real jam on whole grain toast is filling and fun and also REAL. You don't have to eat like a rabbit to eat healthier. Explore the shades of gray.

• • •

I ate my Minty Fudge Brownie Bite in the car on the way home from my meeting with Laura Lea. It was sweet in a different way than a traditional brownie, but so much more satisfying and filling. I'm not going to lie. It wasn't a Snickers bar. The sweet flavor from the dates was subtler, but in combination with the nuts and cocoa, I could taste it better, if that makes sense. It satisfied me without hitting me over the head with a hysterical need for more.

Years ago I would have liked the taste, but I would have been counting calories in my head from the nuts and coconut oil. *Too fatty!* And then I would have spent the next hour pacing around, hungry and frustrated, and eventually made my way to the corner store for a Snickers bar. It never would have occurred to me to eat three or four of her healthy brownie bites to curb the craving and fill up my stomach with food I could use. I was too busy starving and rebounding. I wish I had given myself the chance to make that adjustment back then. It would have saved me a lot of grief. It takes a little while for our brains and taste buds to adjust to the flavors of unpackaged, real food, but not as long as you might think, especially if it's genuinely good.

FOOD THAT FEEDS US

We—as individuals and as a society—have become disconnected from our food at the source. We don't think much about what farmers are up to or what the corporations that package and frankenstein our food are up to either. We are accustomed to buying everything shrink-wrapped with epic amounts of sugar and salt added. We're used to eating dead food out of boxes and bags, and it's killing more than just our stomach linings. It's killing our ambition and destroying our ability to learn and grow.

As the *Harvard Business Review* tells us, "Food has a direct impact on our cognitive performance, which is why a poor decision at lunch can derail an entire afternoon."[4] Sugary and fatty foods throw our bodies and brains into slow motion. They make us sluggish, and when we're sluggish, we lose our swagger. We need good fuel to keep our swagger in shape.

I'm no gardener. Notice a trend? I'm not much into hands-on mastery of growing and making my own food. We don't all have it in us to grow vegetables or experiment in the kitchen all day, but we can support those who do (and ourselves) by purchasing their products, trying their recipes, and following their lead every chance we get. The benefits rub off on us over time.

I recognize that the health and well-being of my gut and brain depend on the meticulous, hard work of people with their hands in the dirt, and I have mad appreciation for them. The providers of pesticide-free fruits, vegetables, and grains; sustainably caught seafood; hormone-free, grass-fed, and free-range meat and dairy; and recipes to put it all together are magicians as far as I'm concerned. They have a lot to teach us, not the least of which is that it's okay to open a can of wild caught salmon and make that the centerpiece of a meal. And it's okay to use frozen spinach, or precooked beans, or eat a nut-and-seed bar from the health food store that's held together with honey. More food. Less chemicals. You don't have to be an organic farmer or an accomplished chef to figure out healthier ways to make your most beloved recipes.

Whether you're choosing red lentil pasta over regular pasta and roasting up a cookie sheet full of frozen broccoli florets like me; clearing your diet of all the clutter and starting over like Rosa; or finding fresh ways to make old favorites like Laura Lea, you can improve what you're eating without a big fuss. It should be good, not miserable.

Food should be rocket fuel for everything else in our lives, a source of connection and pleasure.

The idea is to fill ourselves up with real nutrients so we don't need the empty stuff as much anymore. The emotional triggers that drive us to binge on junk food will still be there. Life won't suddenly become stress-free, but if we're full of good stuff, we won't crave nearly as much of the junk. Over time, real, gratifying food makes us stronger, and the triggers to eat crap get weaker and less frequent.

Fill in the cracks of your diet with whole food any way you can. Let it come up from under you like floodwater on parched Earth, and let yourself be surprised by how good it feels to be full and satisfied. Don't be afraid of healthy fat from avocados and nuts, and don't be afraid of naturally occurring sugar from fruit. Unless you're dealing with a medical condition such as diabetes, these foods are not at the root of any issues you might have with unwanted weight. They are some of the most important tools available to help you find your balance again.

BALANCE

I make the same recipe every Sunday night for my family: individual, thin crust, gluten-free pizzas with spinach, zucchini, red onions, tomato, and veggie "ground beef." The crust is store-bought, and between prep and baking, it takes me under an hour. It's one of just a few recipes I know by heart. I throw things together other nights, but I'm not going to cook every night of the week. I don't want to, and that's okay. The rest of the week I make sure we're eating plenty of fruits and vegetables, even if they're served alongside a can of soup or an organic frozen dinner. The salt in that stuff is beginning to get to me though. My taste buds are changing, and I'm listening.

After watching Laura Lea make her healthy bites, so quickly and easily, I'm questioning my assumption that I can't cook. I'm going to try some of her recipes. We got an Instant Pot recently, too, to mix things up, and the few recipes we've tried so far have me daydreaming about leftovers the following day.

It's time to expand my repertoire. I can get a little bit better each passing week if I keep my eyes and ears open for ways to feed myself and my family whole food that we also happen to like. My husband is on board, too. He got wacky with some skewers on the grill the other night and fed a roomful of our favorite people. "Husband on the grill" is a total cliché, I know, but if that's what he wants to contribute, I am more than happy to cheer him on.

Eating less-processed, more nutritious food might help you lose weight, but that's not the most important point. It will help every other aspect of your life. And it will help you do more good in the world, too, especially if you can achieve a balance, where food means pleasure instead of torture.

Don't give up eating what you love, as long as it makes you feel alive and well. Eat your organic dark chocolate peanut butter cups now and then. Yes, organic. No, not because it's trendy—because it doesn't have ingredients you can't pronounce in it. Yes, it costs more. Yes, you're lucky if you can afford it. And yes, it's worth making healthier versions of your favorite comfort foods a priority in your budget.

Don't be repulsed by food quandaries or by your body. Be repulsed by how junk food and relentless dieting make you feel: foggy, distracted, and desperate.

No more starving. No more challenges. No more fasts. No more pills. Food is not the enemy, and fighting it is making us sick. Food is the remedy that will make us well.

Fill in the Fact

Every time I eat _____,
it makes me feel gross.

My most addictive, unhealthy food habit is _____
_____.

If I try to go a day or two without that habit (circle one):

   (a) I'm a wreck, so I'm going to continue eating it for
       now, *guilt-free.*

   (b) It's not the end of the world, so I'm ready to start
       phasing it out.

A healthier habit or food I could replace it with and still enjoy is

_____.

One healthy food I can easily commit to eating more of is _____

_____.

The next new recipe I'm going to make is _____

_____.

A recipe I love is _____,

and I could make it healthier by changing _____

_____.

 Food has the capacity to hurt or heal. We hold enormous power in our hands every time we lift a bite of food into our mouths.

CHAPTER 7

Alternative Therapies

Okay, you're getting some form of regular exercise. You've made your brownie bites and are feeding your body instead of starving it. You understand the impact of diet and exercise on your ability to show up and get shit done. With stress, we hit the trifecta of well-being. It's time to float—and breathe and pamper and vibe out.

This chapter is a list of fringe and not-so-fringe ways to signal your body to take a load off so you can come back stronger than ever. If you hate lists or don't feel like relaxing, skip it, and move on to Chapter 8. We're going to exit the stratosphere momentarily and return in the next chapter with a flaming, sputtering, meteorite of zero-fucks-left fashion.

This is not medical advice. It's a totally unscientific, layperson's opinion of a few interesting therapies that might help you rejoin your head with your body. This chapter is not meant to be a prescription. It's just a quick list of ways to access your body that you may not have thought of or taken seriously. There is a "skinny wallet version" of each therapy listed as well if you're worried about how much this stuff will cost.

As we've discussed, tension gets stuck in our muscle tissues and nervous systems. There is no shortage of this tension in our modern world, and our bodies physiologically retain information about the stress we endure. Psychotherapy can help us manage stress and anxiety, but we can't always work through physical symptoms by dissecting them intellectually. Sometimes we need to go straight to the body in order to heal.

I've talked a lot about this with Michael Stahl, a licensed massage therapist, Stanford educated lawyer, and founder of the Peregrine Center, a clinic for therapeutic and holistic bodywork. Michael understands body-held trauma both personally and professionally. His spine was fractured during a hockey game when he was fifteen years old, leading to years of pain and physical therapy. At thirty-two, his injury resurfaced and crippled him with pain all over again. This time the doctors, nurses, and bodyworkers were so helpful that they inspired him to pursue a career in restorative massage.

On Michael's website, he describes how our bodies respond to stress and emphasizes that those responses, though frustrating, are generally the body's way of trying to protect itself. "Imagine walking down your street, and your neighbor's dog is barking at you aggressively," he writes. "Suddenly, the fence breaks, and the dog attacks you. You hold up your arms to defend yourself, and the dog bites your arm. You have to go to the hospital to get stitches and shots. The next time you see that dog, your body will almost certainly respond with fear and the physiological response typical of the sympathetic nervous system. . . . The dog hasn't attacked you again, but your mind and body remember the scene, understand that this dog is likely to attack, and put you on high alert to protect against another attack—heart rate elevated, muscles tense, and ready to run or fight off an attack as you walk quickly by the fence."[1]

This same mechanism activates in all of our bodies in response to stress about work, relationships, money, and politics. Have you been passed over for a well-deserved promotion? Catcalled on the street lately? Worried about paying your health insurance premiums? Got dumped? Have a long, stressful commute every day? Terrified the world is descending into a cesspool of division and hatred?

We tense up in order to protect ourselves from potential suffering, but the results of that ongoing burden can be devastating. Stressful situations will keep happening. There's no end in sight there. So, occasionally, we would be well-served to step away from our analytical minds and get back into our bodies in balanced ways in order to prevent the stress from overtaking our health and well-being.

A few moments focused on allowing our lungs to breathe and muscles to release can be deeply therapeutic.

We don't have to carry the burden in our bodies. We can't. At least not all the time. If we do, it will make us sick. It will sap our energy. The question is where to turn, how to relieve the stress burrowing its way through our bodies.

Psychotherapy treatments rooted in biology can offer some relief. A treatment called "biofeedback" can be useful for chronic pain, headaches, and anxiety, among other issues.[2] EMDR (eye movement desensitization and reprocessing) is used to help people recover from PTSD or other traumas, and it is also being used experimentally for eating disorders with some success.[3]

Western medicine can help, too. It gets a bad rap sometimes, particularly by believers in alternative medicine, but, for me at least, Western medicine has been a blessing. It has saved me many times: a broken leg, a fractured elbow, and giving birth in a hospital setting where I was most comfortable, just to name a few. It also kept me from falling through the floor with clinical depression in college. Sometimes chemo, MRIs, antibiotics, antidepressants, or talk therapy are exactly what we need. But sometimes letting our minds rest and reconnecting with our physical bodies for a little while are just what the doctor ordered.

Sometimes we just need to remember that *we have bodies*. We have blood pulsing through our veins. Information comes up from below as much as it comes down from above. We need access to sunshine, air, water, and human touch. When we're shut down from physical or emotional pain, hurting or stressed, we tend to curl up and retreat into cocoons. Lockdown.

I'm not suggesting that any of the therapies in this chapter will abruptly change your circumstances or heal your pain, but if you're dealing with ever-present, generalized stress, they might help, and in some cases, they might help a lot. Consider dabbling in something new. Uncurl long enough to see if one of these therapies makes you feel any better.

Physical disobedience requires breaking out of your own status quo so you can find a new normal, and the ways to do that won't look the same for any two people. If you're an intense, take-charge kind of person, maybe your brand of physical disobedience involves sitting back and breathing while you listen to what somebody else has to say over coffee. If you're reserved and gentle, maybe it involves kickboxing.

Albert Einstein wrote, "The most beautiful thing we can experience is the mysterious. It is the source of all true art and all science. He to whom this emotion is a stranger, who can no longer pause to wonder and stand rapt in awe, is as good as dead: his eyes are closed."[4]

Some of what follows might sound strange, but so what? If your knees are jacked up or you can't stop ruminating on school funding or a broken heart, why not give one a try and see what happens?

• • •

Before we continue, a few things to keep in mind:

1. If something is bothering you, get checked out by a doctor. Alternative therapies can be fantastic, but we also need doctors and nurses. Don't take stupid risks. Checkups are important.

2. When looking for bodywork, find referrals. Ask around to see if your friends have tried these

therapies. People are usually happy to share information about treatments that have made them feel better. You can also look for online reviews, and always make sure that any practitioner you visit has the appropriate accreditations or certifications for his or her scope of practice.

3. You should never feel compromised or unsafe doing any kind of therapy or bodywork. You're the only person who knows what feels good or bad to your body. If you find yourself in a situation that feels uncomfortable or if any aspect of your treatment hurts, speak up. You have the right to change your mind or leave at any time if you don't like what's happening.

That said, here we go.

FLOAT

Let's begin in the weird and wonderful world of sensory deprivation floatation tanks. The tanks were originally invented in the 1950s at the National Institute of Mental Health by neuroscientist and psychoanalyst John C. Lilly. He was pals with Timothy Leary and Allen Ginsberg, so you can glean from that whatever you wish. He was wacky, for sure, but that doesn't mean water and space and time to think aren't useful.

The tanks are approximately eight feet long, four feet wide, and four feet tall. They are designed to provide total, immersive darkness and silence. The water is generally ten to twelve inches deep, containing over eight hundred pounds of Epsom salts. The salt allows you to float without any physical strain and keeps your face effortlessly above the surface of the water. The tanks have a door on the front (which cannot be locked) where you can climb in and out, and you can leave it open or cracked if the dark unnerves you. The tanks are usually placed in spa-like rooms with showers, towels, robes, adjustable lighting, and an external door you can (and should) lock for privacy. Typical sessions last from sixty to ninety minutes.

The practice of therapeutic floating is more common in European countries than in the Unites States, and people have been floating in the Dead Sea, the lowest elevation on Earth, for thousands of years. Floating has been shown to decrease pain, anxiety, and inflammation; decrease blood pressure; and optimize blood flow. Emotional and psychological effects are similar to what you might achieve from a period of extended meditation—stress reduction, a sense of well-being, enhanced creativity, and so on.

I went to Float Nashville to check it out.[5] I have mild claustrophobia, so I was a little freaked out at the thought of being in an enclosed space for ninety minutes. But I discovered that since I couldn't see or hear anything, the small space was essentially irrelevant. I took a shower with a lovely rosemary-mint body wash they provided, put waxy silicone earplugs in my ears to keep the water out as instructed, and climbed in. At first, my body felt a little herky-jerky, as if my muscles were trying to hang on, but within a minute or two, I was able to let them rest. Some people have a hard time trusting the salt water to hold up their heads and struggle to release their necks, so the float centers provide thin foam headrests to support the weight of your head as needed. I tried the headrest at first but discarded it shortly. It wasn't necessary, and I wanted total release.

As time passed, my mind let go, too. I stopped wondering how many minutes had passed and how much longer my session would be. I weaved in and out between full consciousness and a state of mind somewhere between sleeping and waking. When fully awake, I was able to move my shoulder in ways I hadn't in nearly a year. The lack of gravitational pull allowed me to float my arm far overhead and play with internal and external rotation that was normally impossible. Hovering at the edge of sleep, my creative mind wandered. Writing ideas intertwined with imaginative ways to help my clients break through plateaus. I think I fell asleep for a short time but can't be sure. At the end, soft music began to play to bring me back to life. I showered again, slathered on a bunch of lotion, dressed, and wandered out of the room wide-awake.

Ninety minutes away from the buzz? Can't hurt. If you hate silence, some places offer music or you can just play something on your phone, though much of the point is to allow your brain space to wander through the void. If you hate darkness, you can leave the lights on. If you hate water, maybe this isn't your thing, but they claim that the salt is great for your hair and skin. You don't even get wrinkly because the salt content is so high.

Skinny wallet version: After dark, fill up your tub with a heavy dose of bath salts. The water should be warm enough to be comfortable, but not hot enough to make you sweat—near body temperature. Leave your phone and computer turned off in another room. Shut off all of the lights, and get in for a long soak with no agenda and no time limit. Practice letting your limbs float, and, if it feels good, use a bath headrest to support your neck. No book, no magazine, nothing but water and darkness. I actually prefer this option to the spa. I can relax better in my own space, but the floatation tanks do offer true isolation and a lot more space to move. Either way, water is healing, and it would do us all good to immerse ourselves more often.

ACUPUNCTURE

Acupuncture is a central practice of Chinese medicine. It has been used in China for over two thousand years to treat pain and normalize body functions. The World Health Organization (WHO) has a list of dozens of health conditions that can be treated with acupuncture.[6] Some of the most common are headaches, stress, depression, insomnia, PMS, digestive problems, sciatica, recovery during cancer treatments, and all sorts of aches and pains (particularly back and joint pain).

Nobody knows exactly how or why acupuncture works, but through an increasing number of clinical studies, it does seem to work. WHO reports, "Some of these studies have provided incontrovertible scientific evidence that acupuncture is more successful than placebo treatments in certain conditions. For example, the proportion of chronic pain relieved by acupuncture is generally in the range 55–85%, which compares favourably with that of potent drugs (morphine helps in 70% of cases) and far outweighs the placebo effect (30–35%)."

The procedure is totally safe and free of significant side effects. The worst I have ever heard about is minor bruising at an insertion site. Licensed acupuncturists always use sterile, disposable needles that come individually wrapped, and they go to school for three to four years in addition to completing between two hundred and eight hundred hours of clinical practice before becoming accredited. Requirements vary by state, but it is a serious and well-regulated practice. When you go in for treatment, they will ask a series of questions about your overall health, check your pulse, and probably look at your tongue. The tongue apparently tells them all sorts of things about how your body is functioning.

Acupuncture can be administered privately or in a community setting. Private treatments might require removing some of your clothes and lying on a table in a private room, much like you would for a massage. These sessions generally last for a predetermined amount of time according to what your practitioner deems appropriate, usually between thirty and ninety minutes, and cost anywhere from $75 to $150 per treatment.

In a community setting, a large, quiet room with soothing light and music or white noise is set up with a number of recliners, comfortable chairs, or cots. In this case, you stay fully clothed but roll up your pants and sleeves to allow the acupuncturist access to your forearms and lower legs. You can generally kick back with a blanket and stay as long or as briefly as you like. It is my understanding that Chinese medicine dictates that it's important to sit with needles in for at least fifteen to twenty minutes, so I shoot for at least thirty. Treatments in a community setting are often based on a pay-what-you-can structure, ranging between $15 and $40 per treatment.

Once you are settled in either scenario, tiny, sterile needles are inserted into various parts of your body aligning with energy meridians that are believed to run throughout the body carrying qi (pronounced "chee") aka "life force energy." Yep, life force energy. Again, nobody knows why this stuff works, and odds are you are not going to be able to figure it out on your own, so you might as well go with the flow, literally.

Einstein again: "It follow[s] from the special theory of relativity that mass and energy are both but different manifestations of the same thing—a somewhat unfamiliar conception for the average mind."[7] I, for one, definitely have an average mind in comparison to the mad genius with the crazy white hair, so if he says my body is one big coagulation of energy, I'm buying it.

According to Acupuncture.com, "One of the most important concepts of Chinese medicine is that of natural balance. . . . According to this theory, life takes place in the alternating rhythm of yin and yang. . . . Day gives way to night, night to day. . . . the moon waxes and wanes, the tides come in and go out; we wake and sleep, breathe in, breathe out. Yin/Yang . . . are an inseparable couple. Their proper relationship is health. . . . When such a proper balance of forces exists, the body has achieved a healthy circulation of the life force qi."[8]

I have had amazing acupuncture treatments and not so amazing ones. I have left appointments feeling like I could float down the street, and I have left others feeling poked and prodded. The difference has a lot to do with the acupuncturist, his or her bedside manner and level of experience, and my state of mind at the moment. The needles don't usually hurt. I have had some sting a bit going in, but any negative sensations disappear within a minute or two. If a needle is uncomfortable, you can always ask that it be moved or taken out entirely.

The best part of acupuncture is the nap that typically ensues after the needles are inserted. There are working theories that the needles calm the central nervous system, allowing patients to relax. You can't argue with sleep. For more information, check out a pamphlet-sized book called *Why Did You Put That Needle There?* by Andy Wegman. It's on Amazon.com for $8.

Skinny wallet version: Search online for "acupressure point charts." Acupressure uses the same theories as acupuncture but doesn't break the skin. The pressure points often closely align with trigger points used in Western massage. They can be fun to experiment with while hanging out with a friend or a lover. Just make sure you're relaxed, and don't press hard enough to hurt yourself. If anything feels funky, stop. Also, look into community acupuncture in your local area. Prices are usually much lower than private treatments, and the experience can be just as helpful.

REIKI

About a year after having my son, I was having a lot of trouble with my neck. It was seizing up regularly. Most of the time, I was able to continue with my regular life, but about every three months, the muscles would lock down completely, leaving me incapable of lifting my arm, turning my head, or transitioning from standing to lying down or the other way around. When this happened, I was bedbound for several days. The problem had been ongoing for several years while I saw a chiropractor without making progress, and it got worse while I was pregnant and the following year.[9] After enduring yet another flare-up, in the middle of a particularly awful night, I bought a Groupon for a sixty-minute massage at a local new age bookstore/crystal shop. I was low on cash and in need of relief.

I didn't have high hopes going into the treatment room. It was upstairs in a rickety old house with the gift shop below. Isaac, my therapist for the day, was about my age. It turned out he had a son born just a few days after mine, so we commiserated about mutual fatigue. I told him about the neck pain as well as some recurring nerve pain in my hip. After we talked, he left the room. I got undressed, lay face down on the table under a soft sheet and blanket, and waited.

When Isaac came back in the room and gently placed his hands on my neck, I won't say I wept with tears of joy, but I nearly did. It was unlike any other experience I have ever had. His hands radiated heat. Before pulling out any oils or lotions, before digging into my trapezius or rhomboid muscles, he held his hands still and let the heat sink into my body. The muscles, so tight that I could barely function, began to release before he ever moved.

From there, he gave me a typical Swedish massage, following the call and answer of each muscle group from the back of my ears to the bottom of my feet. He was a talented massage therapist, a lucky break for me, but something else was happening, too.

At the end of the massage, on my back this time, he slid his hands under my neck and held them there for at least five minutes. The heat from his hands transferred through my skin, into my back, and shot down both sides of my spine all the way to my tailbone. I laughed out loud. It was so palpable that it was comical. If this person, whom I had never met before, could move heat around in my body like some kind of energy wizard, I was going to have a hard time taking myself too seriously in the future. This was a glorious manipulation of muscle and heat and healing that made no sense, but whatever it was, I wanted more of it.

Isaac was doing Reiki that day, a healing technique I had heard of over the years but didn't really understand. In my early twenties, I dated a massage therapist who was studying Reiki, but that relationship ended in such a mess that when I dismissed the guy, I dismissed Reiki, too.

The International Center for Reiki Training tells us, "Reiki is a Japanese technique for stress reduction and relaxation that also promotes healing. It is administered by 'laying on hands' and is based on the idea that an unseen 'life force energy' flows through us. . . . Reiki treats the whole person including body, emotions, mind and spirit creating many beneficial effects that include relaxation and feelings of peace, security and wellbeing."[10]

There's that "life force energy" again. Reiki relies on the same qi as acupuncture, so if you're not buying into that, you're probably not buying into this. We're getting vibey here, but bear with me.

I began booking sessions with Isaac once a month, and my neck never seized up again. It would begin tweaking out, but if I got to him in time, he could head it off at the pass. I saved a ton of money by quitting the chiropractor. Isaac saved his sanity by quitting the place with the gift shop to work on his own practice, and I referred him to friends and clients, many of whom had similar experiences to mine. (Note: This is not to say that chiropractic care doesn't work in general. It just wasn't helping me in this situation.)

Isaac uses Reiki in combination with massage, as do many massage therapists, but you will also find people who practice Reiki exclusively.

As far as licensing, things get fuzzy when it comes to Reiki. States generally do not license Reiki practitioners because, in theory, it can be administered without ever touching a person. To touch your body, many states require a practitioner to be a licensed massage therapist. However, with informed consent, many people administering Reiki will cup your head or neck in their hands, touch your feet, or other areas as requested (my shoulder, for instance). The only clothes you should ever have to remove for a (nonmassage) Reiki session are your socks and shoes. Rates are roughly equivalent to massage, ranging from $60 to $100 for an hour.

I tried Reiki *without* massage as part of my own practice of physical disobedience. As a proponent of evidence-based science, I was always skeptical of "energy work," but my own experiences and those of my friends and clients have opened my mind over time. One nononsense friend told me that she sought out Reiki after a year of feeling physically and emotionally out of whack after a major loss in her life. She described the session this way. "I felt physical shifts in my body, most notably in the crown of my head, like one might experience a shift in sound when their ears pop, as if space was flooding in. Another obvious sensation was vibration in my hands. It was noticeable in the beginning, enough to need to shift my hands or wiggle them a little, but it became more obvious—so much so, that I felt as if I couldn't move or control the stiffening. It wasn't painful, just a very dominate sensation that would shift from a ripple to extremely fast and warm. When I left the session, I felt open and lighter, like there had been a muddiness that was sifted out."

Lying on the table during my own Reiki session, I watched dappled light dancing behind my closed eyelids and thought, *Ahhh, I could get used to this.* I squinted one eye to peek at the Reiki dude holding his hands above my head and heart. I was resting quite nicely when my shoulder began to throb. Normally, lying still like that, it would not bother me at all, but it felt like the pain was trying to go somewhere and getting stopped, down by my elbow and up through my collarbone. It was so intense I would qualify it as painful, not scary pain but notable enough that I had to bend my arm and place my hand on my stomach to manage the feeling, and eventually it subsided. When I stood up after the hour-long treatment, I had a sense of balance that felt almost disconcerting. It was as if the places in my body that I hold close in a perpetual state of protection (this hip just so, my head tilted a touch to the left, etc.) all released into neutrality. I don't know another way to describe it other than to say that it felt like the boundaries of my body were softer, less contained.

Maybe it was an hour spent resting. Maybe it was a placebo effect of some kind. At the very least, the two greatest promises of Reiki were delivered in full—relaxation and a sense of well-being—and that was enough for me.

Skinny wallet version: Evidence abounds, even in Western culture, that the boundaries between body, mind, and spirit are blurry, and we often express that interchange with our hands. When we attend church or yoga class, we press the palms of our hands together over our chests to center our hearts and minds. We hold hands with loved ones to feel closer in times of love and grief. When people pray for someone who is ailing, they place their hands on or near the person they are praying for. The blind are able to perceive people and objects in their immediate vicinity with heightened spatial awareness, functioning at or near the capacity of a sighted person, but when those objects are farther away, they become disoriented.[11] And when my son skins his knee and burrows into my arms, the only thing that takes the pain away is the feeling of my hands rubbing his back or holding firmly near (but not at) the site of the injury.

These ancient customs speak to the intuitive sense that healing can be conferred through human hands. We can all do this for each other with no training whatsoever. If you or a friend is hurting, with permission, in a peaceful room, spend some time holding your hands on or near the part of the body where it hurts, or if the pain is emotional, hold them up around the crown of the head or over the heart. You can't go wrong spending time together focused on rest and healing.

MASSAGE

If "life force energy" is a step too far for you, massage is a version of healing touch you can probably get your head around. Relaxed muscles and healthy blood flow are good things for everybody. Also, massage is used extensively in sports medicine, and if it's recommended for Lindsay Vonn and Michael Phelps, it's got to be good for the rest of us, too, right?

It is my sincere hope that everyone reading this passage has had a massage in his or her lifetime, preferably within the last few months. If that is not the case for you, put the book down, and ask your friends where they go. Make an appointment as soon as possible, and go lie down on a table under the skillful hands of someone who is trained to help relieve your body of stress. Everyone can benefit from healing touch. Even animals respond to it. Give your dog or cat a massage and watch what they do—roll over, purr, stretch, yawn, and release.

Massage can take many forms. The most common is *Swedish* massage, which is all about relaxation. It can be administered with a light or firm touch and often involves aromatherapy oils mixed with oil or lotion. *Hot stone* massages are also super-relaxing. They oil you up and rub smooth, round, hot stones over your aching muscles. Oily, hot, and fabulous. *Shiatsu* is the one where they pound on your muscles rhythmically. It makes me want to go, "ahhhheeeeeeooooooh" to hear the sound vibrate in my chest cavity like a little kid.

More intense methods include deep tissue, trigger point, and myofascial work. *Deep tissue* massage digs into knots or adhesions in your muscles to help them let go. *Trigger point* targets small areas of tight muscle tissue that can refer pain to other areas. *Myofascial* work can be done by a massage therapist or a physical therapist. It involves slow, sustained pressure to break up or elongate fascia, a weblike tissue that runs between our skin, muscles, and all of our organs. It holds everything together but can clump up, causing pain and stiffness.

If a massage hurts to the point where you want to recoil from it, it's probably a step too far, though in some prescribed medical settings, pushing through the pain can be useful. Either way, you always have the right to ask your therapist to lighten up.

Any massage therapist should be able to work with you fully or partially clothed if you like, but I highly recommend getting naked if you're comfortable with it. You should always be able to dress and undress in private before and after a massage, and the majority of your body should always be draped with a sheet. The therapist will unwrap each arm, leg, back area, and so on, as needed. Private parts should never see the light of day. If you have a bleeding disorder or acute injuries or wounds, check with a doctor before seeing a massage therapist. For everyone else, if you haven't ever had a massage or haven't had one in a long time, go get one as often as time and money allow.

Touch is an essential human need. Biologically, massage can improve muscle function and return homeostasis to various body systems. Psychologically and spiritually, it knows no bounds. We are not meant to live without touch. Give yourself an hour when you can. You won't regret it.

Skinny wallet version: The beauty of massage is that anyone can do it. Swap backrubs or foot massages with a friend. If you are alone or truly can't afford a massage, you can get various rollers and massage wands that can be used solo to access and release sore spots. You can even find a nail salon with a massage chair and let the vibration take you away while you get your pedicure done. But if at all possible, get a full-body massage from a trained therapist. Skip pedicures or fancy coffee for a few weeks to save up for it. Whether from a friend or a professional, human hands make it so much better.

PHYSICAL THERAPY

Physical therapy doesn't get the love it deserves, probably because it's slow. People don't like slow. They want quick results, but our bodies take a long time to build strength, stability, and flexibility. If you're recovering from an injury or surgery or if you have weakness or stiffness that is compromising your ability to function at full steam, PT can be critically important for recovery. I have seen so many people injure and re-injure the same areas of their bodies because they didn't take the time to do the PT exercises prescribed. I know it's boring. I know it's a pain—in fact, physical therapy can be very uncomfortable, and improvements can come at a snail's pace—but if you stick with it, you will set yourself up for a stable, healthy body in the future. Delayed gratification is the norm on this one. Sorry. But it is so, *so* important. Listen to your physical therapist, and follow through at home. It makes a difference.

Skinny wallet version: Physical therapy is frequently covered, at least to some degree, by health insurance if you're lucky enough to have it. Check with your insurer; you might need a doctor's prescription to get started. Once you have gone through the initial course of treatment, if you're making progress, you can usually save some cash by taking many (or all) of the exercises home to keep working on your own. The key is sticking with them. It helps to tie the exercises to a daily ritual you're already doing, like drinking your morning coffee or getting ready for bed. Just make sure you know what you're doing with the stretches or exercises before trying them on your own.

MEDITATION

Last, but maybe most important, is meditation. Here's the thing about meditation: It doesn't have to be about an esoteric practice of silencing your mind. It doesn't require sitting in the lotus position with your hands in gyan mudra (first finger and thumb forming a circle). It can be done walking, washing dishes, sitting in a chair, or in your car.

According to Fadel Zeidan, PhD and associate director of neuroscience at the Wake Forest Center for Integrative Medicine, mindfulness meditation is simply "nonjudgmental awareness of the present moment." In other words, it's a practice of separating painful thoughts or sensations from the emotional and psychological reverberations that amplify them. Your thoughts don't own you. They come; they go; they linger and nag; and then they wander off again. Meanwhile, nothing happened. The universe didn't come screeching to a halt. You survived, and now you're on to the next thing.

According to Dr. Zeidan, the same can be true for physical pain. His studies show that people can use mindfulness meditation to divorce painful physical sensations from dread and fear, thereby reducing their perception of pain by 44 percent. These results are measurably better than the placebo effect of sitting quietly and breathing, at 24 percent reduction of pain, and the effectiveness of a dose of morphine, at 20 percent reduction of pain.[12]

Mindfulness may sound trivial or obscure, but there is hard science to back it up. Meditation isn't necessarily about emptying our minds.

It's about recognizing clutter for what it is and learning how to coexist with it, diminishing its impact rather than magnifying it. It's a powerful form of disobedience if you think about it: *This situation is what it is, and I choose not to amplify it in my mind. It is my choice, and I choose to let it be. And, what do you know, I'm still sitting here, intact and functional.*

If you don't like sitting still, restorative yoga, qi gong, walking, or tai chi are all great ways to physically move your body while getting many of the advantages of meditation. Even sports like swimming, running, or golf offer meditative benefits, especially if you're practicing letting thoughts and feelings come and go, free of baggage, while you're at it. Also, any meditation that gets you outside, adding fresh air and light to the mix, whether sitting or moving, brings you back in contact with the big, old Earth that we're living on—and that is healing in and of itself.

Some purists might not consider these activities to be true meditation. However, they *are* all forms of "ecotherapy," a treatment prescribed by a growing number of doctors and psychotherapists to promote physical and psychological equilibrium without the use of drugs. You can prescribe yourself twenty or thirty minutes a day outdoors and be reasonably confident that it will impact your body and state of mind positively.

All of this is free. No need for a skinny wallet version. You can take classes, of course, but you can also find a ton of information and free instruction online. For seated or walking meditation, check out the Insight Timer app (or hundreds of other available apps) for silent or guided meditations. I like Insight Timer because when you're done, it shows you the hundreds or thousands of people you just meditated with all over the world who were using the timer at the same time as you. It makes you feel a little more connected.

• • •

Most of us know we have lots of options for exercise. It's not too hard to think out of the box athletically. We can climb a rock wall or take karate or ride a bike or take a barre class or play soccer or run marathons or do yoga. It's harder to imagine alternative ways to relieve pain and reduce anxiety, but a little bit of exploration can go a long way.

<><><><><><><><><><><><><><><><><><><><><><><><><><><><><><><><>

Fill in the Fact

The last time I tried a new relaxing treatment was _____
_____.

I love this therapy— _____ —but
don't do it often enough.

I've been going in for _____
treatments for a while, but they don't seem to be helping.

Instead, I would like to try _____
_____.

I will schedule this treatment: _____, by
this date: _____.

<><><><><><><><><><><><><><><><><><><><><><><><><><><><><><><><>

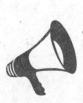

Less stress equals better
choices. Better choices equal
better health. Better health
equals a better life and more
"life force" to get things done.

CHAPTER 8

Fashion

This just in my inbox: J.Lo knows how to make my ponytail "EXTRA" awesome. It's going to be my next "date night hair." Goodie. Also, Stitch Fix wants me to come back, even though I return everything they send me. Not their fault. Mine. I'm picky, and apparently I hate everything that isn't made of jersey cotton. Basically, I'm a fashion Luddite. My life as a personal trainer offers very few requirements for grown-up clothing, so I never learned the tricks. I live in yoga pants, jeans, and cotton skirts. I try to wear shirts that button up sometimes, but I can't breathe; so I strip them off and leave them in a pile on the floor in exchange for a loose tank top.

I stand in awe of my friends who make real fashion choices, who throw together a jumpsuit with a cropped jacket and a head wrap for a night out. I may not know much about fashion, but I can certainly appreciate the power of it. The ways we choose to adorn ourselves in public can make or break our confidence, and that can have wide social reverberations. Fashion can help illuminate who we are or it can make us feel like walking automatons.

Feminist fashion can't really be defined. It is as unique as we are, but when I think about the potential for fashion to support our true selves, our activism and ambitions, two core values seem obvious: freedom of choice and freedom of expression. Too often, we rely on clothes to obscure our bodies, to pin and tuck them into shape, rather than choosing outfits based on what liberates us for work and play. When we follow trends regardless of how they suit us or give up altogether out of sheer exhaustion, we do ourselves a disservice. Both of those choices make us lesser, not greater versions of ourselves.

Most of the time, my primary ambition is to find ways to appear functionally groomed without compromising too much time and energy. But increasingly, I'm hoping to achieve more than that. I'm hoping to discover and amplify my confidence and sense of adventure, whatever that might look like. That goes for hair, makeup, clothes—the whole thing.

HAIR

I have found that hair is a particularly direct way to communicate to the world that I am either polished and ready to go or vying for a starring role in a documentary about insomnia and hoarding. Sometimes cutting it all off seems like the best way to handle this dilemma, but the few times I've done that, I look just as haggard as before and not at all like myself. So I let it grow and play around with various gels and wands. My African American friends tell me that the decision about how to wear their hair has even further-reaching repercussions for them. The choices they make have personal and societal implications I can only begin to imagine.

Hair is so closely tied to identity, but I never fully understood how significantly my hair reinforces (or undermines) my sense of self until I talked with Stephanie Williams Caillabet, a master wig maker in Austin, Texas.

Stephanie got her start at the LA Opera and Jim Henson's Creature Shop, and she has worked on dozens of movies and TV shows, making wigs and doing special effects makeup for *The Cat in the Hat*,

The Grinch, Planet of the Apes, Six Feet Under, Outer Limits, Charmed, Nip/Tuck, and *Spiderman II,* among others. But Stephanie's Hollywood resume is the least interesting thing about her. Far more interesting is the work she has done in the second half of her career.

After moving to Austin over a decade ago, she was asked to make a wig for a powerful, female lobbyist who was undergoing chemotherapy treatments for breast cancer while pregnant. Stephanie told me, "She wanted to hide the fact that she was pregnant and going through chemo at the same time because she was afraid people would think (wrongly) that she was killing her baby, and it would damage her career. She wanted to bide her time until she had the baby. The day I put on her wig was the first time I got into the medical side of wig making. I put the wig on her, and she grabbed her husband's hand and said, 'Oh my God, I think I'm going to be able to do this.' Until then, I had no idea she was nervous or insecure. She's just a fierce, awesome woman. They both started crying, and I thought, 'Well, this is what I'm going to do for the rest of my life.'"

Since then, Stephanie has made a career of helping women who are dealing with cancer, alopecia (hair loss due to immune or hormonal problems), trichotillomania ("hair-pulling" disorder), or any other kind of female hair loss. "With chemo patients, we have big head shaving parties here with champagne and photos. Those are fun," she says.

A lot of her clients come in saying that they only want a wig for backup and plan to get by with hats and scarves, "but they end up wearing them all the time. You can't really hide that you're bald under a scarf or hat, and people look at you like you're sick. You could be having the best day ever, a super great day and not feel like crap at all, but people will look at you like you're dying. It just throws you back down. So it's important to them to look like themselves, to make it really natural. It gives them their sexy back, their confidence."

Stephanie repeated several times during our conversation, "People want to look like themselves." As I thought about that, I realized that I have very little idea what that means for me. I wear what's expedient. Most of the time, I do my hair in ten seconds after getting out of the shower with a palm full of styling cream. This was a groundbreaking concept to me. We want to look like ourselves! Of course! Wouldn't it be magical if that notion were at the center of every decision about what to wear, rather than stressing about how it looks from the outside?

"It's nobody's business," Stephanie told me. "It's up to each of my clients how they want to battle their disease."

Right? It's up to each of us to decide what hair and clothes and mascara we wear or don't wear. It's nobody's business how any of us want to look, whether undergoing cancer treatments or going on a first date. We're all just trying to feel like ourselves.

I started using this concept as a barometer for every outfit, every pair of shoes, every hairstyle, and every bit of makeup I put on my face—and honestly, it made me feel mischievous. *Does this make me feel like myself?* I couldn't remember the last time my attention was focused on feeling free rather than worried about how I looked from the outside. Maybe that says something sad about me. Maybe I was being vain, and I'm all alone in this breathtaking discovery that fashion should feel like freedom. Anyway, I'm never going back. The coming decades are going to be an entertaining ride in combat boots and color.

Stephanie sets aside 10 percent of her profits to make wigs for kids who can't afford to pay for them. One of her most beloved clients is a nine-year-old girl named Adalia Rose. Adalia has a genetic condition, called "progeria," that causes kids to age rapidly. It affects one in four million people, and life expectancy with the disease is around thirteen years. Stephanie made Adalia's first wig when Adalia was five. "She wanted her mommy's long black hair," Stephanie said. So Adalia's mom shaved her head, and Stephanie made a long, beautiful wig. Since then, she has made several more for her, including one with donations from the Austin Firefighters Association. The most recent is a long, blonde mermaid wig that reaches down "past her butt." Adalia hasn't grown since she was four, and she only weighs around twenty-two pounds. Kids with progeria often require hip replacements and hearing aids. They have strokes, cataracts, and glaucoma. Adalia faces all of these challenges, but she's also a force. She is an internet sensation with fourteen million followers on Facebook.

"She's huge on social media," Stephanie said, "and she wants to be a professional makeup artist. She's got so much sass and attitude, such a personality in such a little body." Stephanie asked Adalia why she likes to wear her wigs. "They make me feel prettier! And famous!" she said. And pretty and famous, she is. She is also irrepressible and very much herself. We could all take a lot of inspiration from people like Adalia. Her body doesn't fit anybody's mold of traditional beauty, but she has found a spectacular beauty all her very own.

Stephanie works in the "beauty" industry, but the beauty she's creating isn't reliant on perfection. In fact, quite the opposite, this kind of beauty unfolds in the hearts and minds of her clients when they are able to return to normal, back to themselves, as they want to be. "It's so amazing to change somebody's life like that," she said, "to take them from 'I can't do this, and I'm having a hard time waking up in the morning' to 'Holy crap, let's go to Target!' I couldn't be more in love with what I do."

We all need to find our own personal template for Holy crap, let's go to Target! It's the opposite of Screw this. I hate everything. I'm staying home.

So what does that look like for you? What does it look like for me?

After talking with Stephanie, I decided to grow my hair out again. I cut it to shoulder length a few years ago because I wanted to look smart. I thought that if I kept it long, it would look immature, like I was trying to be a teenager or something, but when I sat back to think about what feels easy and authentic to me, long is it, for now anyway. Shorter hair didn't make me look smart. It made me look awkward because I *felt* awkward.

And in my wardrobe? I want romance and comfort. I want understated, long, feminine lines in earthbound colors with a whisper of detail. I want flexible, breathable fabric that offers some semblance of structure and shape.

I think.

Or maybe I don't. Maybe I want something else entirely.

CLOTHES

Sandhya Garg is a fashion designer who appeared on Season 13 of *Project Runway*. She won two challenges, including the first one of the season, and was famously maligned by some her fellow designers, two of them calling her by a series of unmentionable racial slurs.

Sandhya is an Indian immigrant. She graduated from the London College of Fashion and has worked at Alexander McQueen, Gucci, Liberty London, and Alice Temperley. She has shown at New York Fashion Week and her brand has been featured in *Marie Claire*, *Elle*, and *Cosmopolitan*. She refers to her design sensibility as "maximalism." She uses explosive color and print in modern, innovative ways. Some of her clothes are high fashion, beyond what some of us would want to pull off, but the vast majority of her work is designed for real women in real situations, with a splash of *holy shit*.

"My Indian heritage includes a lot of beautiful textiles, embroidery, and fiber crafts," she told me. "I am proud of where I come from, and it has formed my design aesthetic. India is all about beautiful, bright, vibrant colors. It's a warm, love-filled country with a lot of folklore and mythology. My inspiration comes from my life. I think we see so much beauty around us, and sometimes we just want to wrap ourselves in it. I design for those women, regular women in all shapes and sizes. I encourage them to take risks yet be comfortable. In the end, if they're not comfortable, there is no point taking a risk."

Wrapping ourselves in beauty? This woman is speaking my language. I have absolutely no idea what I'm "supposed to be wearing" this season, but whatever it is, it's too narrow. Wrapping myself in beauty is the only rule I need.

"Feminism in fashion is all about defining who you are through your clothes," Sandhya said, "owning your own style and not letting other people's views define you. I think women of all shapes, sizes, ages, and ethnicities are beautiful. My influences come from different people, architecture, cultural vibe, all the energy that makes us happy. Some might say they are 'carrying sunshine in their pocket.' My inspiration is about wearing sunshine. For me, fashion is more than just design, it's a lifestyle choice and a social channel to talk about important issues."

Following the "rules" of fashion has lassoed us into a noose of acceptable female behavior and appearances. It binds our bodies. It knits our legs together and prevents us from taking up space. It compels us to obey.

What happens to a female attorney at the highest levels of a Dallas law firm who wears clogs to work because they make her feel more grounded? Does she get passed over for promotion because she's not as tall as she might be, because her hips aren't tilted back and her chest protruding just enough? Maybe. Or does she do her work more effectively and take the lead in crucial investigations? I imagine it depends on what *she* thinks of her clogs. If they make her feel dull and flat-footed, she'll retreat into the walls. But if they make her feel capable and dynamic—while her superiors are worrying about her unwillingness to conform—she is busy taking over the firm.

Clogs and pumps are equally feminist, as long as they set us free. The question is, do your fashion choices make you feel like *Damn these pants are tight*, or do they make you feel like *Hell yeah, here I go!*

There is a difference between how an item of clothing looks in a catalog and how it feels on your body. By listening to what feels right on and around your body, you can make choices that make you want to do a happy dance, and if it freaks some people out, that's their problem, not yours. Let everyone else travel lockstep in whatever obligatory outfits work for them. You might have to follow some basic rules of propriety at work, but there are always ways to make your outfits your own with fabrics and colors you love and accessories that make you want to tell everyone where you got that killer necklace.

The hard part is figuring out what makes you feel *both beautiful and at ease*, and that task is especially difficult if you're not happy with the shape of your body. So make a game of it. Head into the dressing room like Erykah Badu or Kesha. Jeans that are cut just right can make your bootie feel *magnifico*. And if you can find a great tailor, you can buy big and take anything in around the curves. The number on the tag is meaningless, and alterations are miraculous. I don't take my clothes in for alterations often enough, but I'm about to get on that.

UNDER THE CLOTHES

Tig Notaro knows more than most about throwing people off with a controversial fashion choice. She is a comedian who became famous in the wake of her mother's sudden death and her own cancer diagnosis in 2012. Just days after being diagnosed, she performed a set at Largo in Los Angeles, California. She kicked off the show with a cheerful, friendly greeting, telling the crowd, "Good evening, hello! I have cancer, how are you? Hi, how are you? Is everybody having a good time? I have cancer. How are you?" And the crowd lost it. They didn't know what to think. Clearly there was discomfort in the audience, but the overwhelming responses were laughter, awe, and relief—the relief of being in a room with someone who is willing to set aside all pretense to be ruthlessly real. It was scary and funny at the same time.

Three years later, post–double mastectomy and still very much alive, Tig took that ruthless honesty to the next level by removing her shirt onstage in the middle of a performance that was being recorded for her HBO special, *Tig Notaro: Boyish Girl Interrupted*. She performed the rest of the set topless.

Tig has a habit of bulldozing societal expectations.

When I saw the video of her standing on stage during that performance—smooth, bare-chested and carrying on with the comedy like nothing out of the ordinary was happening—I was elated and excited and confused. Her body looked strange and fresh, like a barely pubescent teenage boy on summer vacation, and she was just doing her thing, continuing on with the show with a glint in her eye. This was a new and different kind of openness from anything I had ever seen before. It was defiant and groundbreaking but utterly non-combative. She was just Tig, with a shrug and a wink, and I longed to know what that kind of freedom felt like.

The shock factor wasn't about the nudity. I wasn't sure if this even qualified as nudity. Is a man on stage with his shirt off considered "nude"? There were no breasts anywhere in sight, no nipples, just a body and some good jokes. The strangeness of where that fell in our cultural norms hit me like a bullet train. How can it be that going topless with amputated breasts takes a person from doing something illegal or "pornographic" to being totally acceptable?

Does this mean that Tig gets to wear swim trunks at the beach now? Can she play Frisbee in shorts at the park with her shirt off like a guy? I imagine she could. When I'm at the YMCA pool in July, the last thing I want on my body is a tight, bralike structure. I want to understand why it's the end of the world if I take my top off at the pool and roll over on my back to enjoy the sun, but if I chop my boobs off, *all good*!

Tig's autobiography is titled *I Am Just a Person*, and it's true. She is just a person, just like us. She is a person who has taken risks, time and again, to stay true to herself, and we are the benefactors of those choices. When she took off her shirt on national TV, she shed daylight on millions of women who have undergone breast cancer treatments and mastectomies, but, really, she was speaking to all of us. At least in my eyes, she was saying, *Hey! Hi. This is just a body. We all have bodies, and isn't it silly how weird we are about how they look? My body is still here, and this is how it looks, and I'm good with that.*

With one gutsy fashion choice, Tig Notaro cut me loose to let my body be exactly what it is.

I think a lot of us feel like our bodies are an affront to the outside world. We assume because we aren't easy on the eyes like underwear models that we're committing some sort of sin just by being present with thicker bellies and thighs. So we hide and twist and cower to make ourselves less offensive.

Being where you are—head on, wearing clothes you like, and allowing your body, as it is, to be part of the moment at hand—is an act of defiance. Try it. You might like it. It's a power trip. Dudes do it all the time. Why shouldn't we?

YOUR BODY, YOUR CLOTHES, YOUR WAY

Growing up, I felt my throat catch every time someone asked me what kind of music I liked. What if they didn't like the same as me? What if they thought I wasn't cool? What if my taste in music proved beyond a shadow of a doubt that I wasn't cool and I didn't even know it? You couldn't have paid me a thousand dollars to DJ a basement party. I was way too stressed out about whether my flannel was too grungy or not grungy enough.

Trying to keep up with the cool kids leads to a tippy-toe existence where everything we do involves waiting to see which way the wind is blowing before we jump in with an opinion. But phony clothes, workouts, diets, musical inclinations, reading lists, hairstyles—or any other choices that don't feel right to us—are keeping us in fake, bobblehead, alternative realities where everything we genuinely care about suffers.

Following your gut is scary, but following someone else's gut is just plain sad. It's vacant. If we tell ourselves (and everybody else) little lies about what kind of fashion works for us, those falsehoods create a million little cuts to our stability and happiness.

Play the music you like. Wrap yourself in sunshine. Shave your head, or let your hair down. Adalia Rose wouldn't think twice about her fashion choices, and neither should you.

Wear what makes you feel like yourself.

Bogus clothes and hairstyles aren't doing any of us any good.

Who are we trying to impress anyway? We want to attract lovers and friends—but do we want to be with people who approve of our awkward, on-trend makeup and heels, or do we want to be with people who love us for who we are? The only fail-safe way to engage with friends, jobs, and partners that fit well is to check back in with who you are and dress in ways that feel uplifting—try a new style or dig deeper into the ones you already know and love.

Would part of me like to get a pixie cut to find out what it feels like to be free of this mass of frizz? Absolutely. But a larger, louder part of me loves my sloppy, long hair. It keeps me warm in the winter.

And would I go boobs out at the pool all summer if it wouldn't get me arrested? Affirmative. But it would, so I won't. There are, of course, legal constraints on how we dress our bodies, but not that many. Keep the privates covered. Fine. But beyond that, your choices are your own.

I'm eager to explore the hues of sunshine color embodied by Sandhya Garg's designs. And someday maybe I'll chop off my hippy hair and donate it to Stephanie, but, for now, I'm hanging on. It makes me more myself. Maybe J.Lo can show me some fancy ways to fix it, if I ever get around to opening that email.

Wear what you want, when you want. It's your body and your prerogative. What we can't do anymore is squeeze ourselves into somebody else's sense of style and decorum.

Life is too short for that, and there's no such thing as one size fits all.

◇◇

Fill in the Fact

I like my hairstyle (circle one):

Yes   No

If I took a risk with my hair I would _____

_____.

I feel comfortable and happy in my clothes (circle one):
  Yes   No

A style I wear all the time but am tired of is _____

_____.

A style I'd like to try is _____

_____.

A fashion choice I love but don't wear because of insecurity is

_____.

My dressing room alter ego is _____

_____.

Wear what makes you
feel like yourself.

CHAPTER 9

Motherhood

I might need to have my sanity checked for wandering into the topic of motherhood here, but screw it. The truth shall set us free. This chapter is dedicated to any mom who feels like she is falling short; to fence-sitters who are unsure about taking the leap into motherhood; to women who have lost a child in a miscarriage or stillbirth; and, more broadly, to every woman who has ever nurtured another living creature's spirit at her own expense—because they are moms, too, regardless of whether or not they have ever physically given birth.

Motherhood is about love, and—biological moms or not—we are all the same in our love and our capacity for outreach. The sacrifices required and the benefits achieved by caring for others are the forces that keep humanity afloat. Motherly love of any sort teaches us what we are capable of.

I'm no expert on how mothering is supposed to be done, so please take everything I say about this topic with a grain of salt, especially with regard to actual human children. I haven't read the books. I didn't grow up wanting to be a mother. I didn't have any sort of clock ticking in my twenties or thirties. Mostly, I just wanted to be able to sleep in for the rest of my life—but that wasn't meant to be.

I met a guy, and we had a kid, and now he's our little man. So that's awesome, and also demanding and mind-boggling. I have no idea what I'm doing. But becoming a mom taught me more than I ever could have imagined about disobedience, about how to go my own way and stop giving so much of a damn what anybody else thinks about how I'm supposed to look or behave.

When I did become a mom, I continued to avert my eyes from all of the shoulds and shouldn'ts. *Nothing to see here!* I asked for all the drugs while giving birth. My son had a tied tongue that made breast-feeding impossible without cutting it, so I pumped furiously for two months before playing my sanity card and switching to Walmart Organic Formula. I let him cry it out at six months so he could sleep through the night, and now he eats pressed fruit leather several times a day instead of real fruit. He is five years old. I read to him every night, but I don't review flash cards or do word problems before bed.

Let the slings and arrows fly if you must. I have no interest in arguing with anyone about any of those choices.

The only thing I know for a fact about motherhood is that no mom should have to jump through anyone else's mommy hoops—assuming, of course, that the kids are safe and loved. We're all just doing our best, and a little kindness (toward ourselves and each other) goes a long way. Honesty is the best we can do. So here goes.

FUEL ON THE FIRE

I was scared to death to be a mom. From the outside, it looked like a vortex into which all ambition and self-determination would be forever suffocated. I felt that way up to and beyond the moment I lay my son in the crib for the first time—a tightrope walk between awe and panic.

Though I never imagined myself as a mom, when the time came, I did decide to do it on purpose. It wasn't an accident. I did it in blatant defiance of my own terror. I figured if I could face down my greatest fear and emerge maybe even better off, I could handle anything. I was playing a game of Russian roulette when I had spontaneous sex that peaceful, winter, Wednesday afternoon. If I became pregnant and managed to find joy in what lay beyond that, I won. If not, I was in for a lifelong challenge.

As my belly grew, when asked about my "birth plan," I used to say that I felt as if I had made an appointment with the mafia to be beaten and disemboweled. Pregnancy and birth signified a loss of control and obliteration of my identity so complete that I genuinely doubted my ability to survive. I doubted my body, and I doubted my mind.

Before making this questionable decision, I believed that freedom (and thereby, happiness) was achieved by a lack of responsibility—and let me be clear, I still very much enjoy a lack of responsibility, particularly beachside. But what I didn't realize was that instead of breaking my spirit, motherhood would make me reassess who I want to be and prioritize what I have to offer.

The motherhood I feared was heavy with burden and boredom, but what I discovered—and what I found in some of my friends who took the same path—is that motherhood has the capacity to be a means to freedom, an urgent push to spur us on toward greater realization of ourselves rather than a subjugation of our needs to those of our children.

The first year of motherhood is, without question, a time for recovery and finding a new rhythm. It's a balancing act with cereal in our hair and sharp knives perched precariously on the top shelf. But beyond the initial shock, having a kid can be fiercely liberating, reconnecting us with our greatest ambitions and the extraordinary power of our bodies at work.

My gentle, cautious, lanky, little boy's stability and fulfillment in life hinges not on my being able to coddle him into adulthood. With a loving, reliable framework around him, it hinges on his parents continuing to be whole people: growing, failing, changing, and being available most of the time, but not all of the time.

I'll do everything in my power to make sure he has all the food, exercise, shelter, love, and education he needs, but it's also my duty to help him understand that he is not the center of the universe. Empathy. Other people's needs matter as much as his own, and there is a lot he can do to help fill those needs.

The best example I can set for him is one fueled with fire for living and loving, a life in which I can move and stretch and breathe and give so he can learn to do the same. Motherhood, much to my surprise, turned out to be an incredible blessing. It changed the landscape of my days for sure, but it didn't change the trajectory of who I am or the contributions I hope to make. In fact, by hemming me in, it has driven me to burn brighter.

Motherhood is kerosene on the fire, and my son is the best reason I ever had to live bigger, wider, and stronger.

When we find ourselves, as moms, taking third place, or fourth or fifth, we need to consider what we're doing. We are the examples our kids replicate. If we martyr ourselves for motherhood, we set our little ones at war in their own hearts, in a fierce, confusing battle between selfishness and self-destruction.

We can't be good moms if we don't take care of ourselves. We can't be good caretakers, leaders, or mentors for each other if we can't breathe.

Like they say on the airplane, you have to put your own mask on first. We need to take better care of ourselves, body and soul, so our kids can learn to take better care of *them*selves, too, while finding their own ways to make a difference.

Motherhood seems like the ultimate sacrifice—or that's the story we're sold—but that has not been my experience. Being a mom is definitely the hardest thing I have ever done, but the mother–child relationship feeds and fuels both parties. It's a comedy of errors, a game of Twister where we try to hold each other up by positioning ourselves just the right way. We will certainly fall down in a heap, time and again, piled on top of each other, but at least we'll be in the heap together, staring at the ceiling and waiting for the dog to come lick our faces.

I would never take my decision to become a mom back, not just because I adore my kid (though I do) and not because it's socially unacceptable to regret motherhood (though it is). I wouldn't take that decision back because of what it has taught me about being curious, vulnerable, and driven.

I've learned about my own stubbornness and my nearly pathological need for autonomy because I see those impulses in my son. I've learned how to pick my battles and how to ride the wave of unrelenting change and chaos. I've learned that I'm capable of flying into a rage for stupid reasons if I'm tired and that those rages are terrifying to those around me. They are unacceptable, and the only one who can stop that madness is me. Most important, I've learned that everybody loves his or her kids as much as I love mine. We're all the same, all over the world. Our pride, pain, and frustration are all the same. There is simply no difference between me and a Syrian mom who has lost everything in a cluster bomb—and that sameness is unbearably unfair. All of those lessons have made me a kinder person, and I'm sure there are more lessons to come.

* * *

We are all moms if we choose to be. We are doting mothers to our groups of friends. We are ever-present mothers to every kid that ever gets lost at a concert or on a street corner. We are devoted mothers to our pets. And we are mothers of the modern feminist revolution, owing our roots to Rosa Parks and Elizabeth Cady Stanton. Together, we blink our eyes in disbelief that we "still have to protest this shit."

Our voices need to be heard—legislatively, in PTAs, in the media, and at the helm of Fortune 500 companies. Our perspectives on long-neglected policies that will benefit every living person on earth need to be at the forefront of business and government—not in spite of the time we put in as moms, but because of it.

Men can be incredible caregivers as well. I do not mean to disparage their contributions as fathers of children or of planet Earth, but as women, a different perspective runs through us. Historically, that insight has been marginalized, but the planet would be a safer, more abundant place for both men and women if our positions of power matched our percentage of the population.

According to a report by the Pan American Development Foundation, "Providing girls and women with increased access to education, jobs, healthcare, and other services has a substantial ripple effect, improving not only individual quality of life, but also that of the surrounding community. We know that girls and women multiply the impact of investments by extending the benefits far beyond themselves. They are heads of families, leaders in their communities, business owners, and changemakers."[1] All you have to do is look around at the women in your immediate circle to know that this is true.

We give a damn, and we show up.

FIILING IN THE GAPS

Courtenay Rogers was born in San Diego, California. She was one of two kids born to a naval officer father and a substitute teacher mom. They lived all over the country during her childhood, changing bases every few years to accommodate her father's assignments. As a kid she was a cheerleader, and she loved participating in student government and journalism. While attending the University of Mississippi, she joined the ROTC and was commissioned as a naval officer upon graduation. She served in the US Navy on a guided missile destroyer out of Pearl Harbor and became USS *Hopper* Junior Officer of the Year in 2003 while serving in the Persian Gulf during Operation Enduring Freedom.

Courtenay fell in love and got married when she was twenty-five. Three years later, she gave birth to a baby girl, but by the time her daughter was eighteen months old, the marriage became unsustainable. She left her husband and took the baby to Franklin, Tennessee, where her parents had settled for retirement.

Back in civilian life, Courtney became a technology consultant. In 2014, she and two of her best friends (one of whom is also a single mom) founded Girls to the Moon, a social enterprise company dedicated to "launching confident girls to be their best selves, impact their communities, and create a more inclusive culture."[2]

In 2016, she was recruited by the Democratic Party to run for the Tennessee House of Representatives as a progressive in a deeply conservative county. "I was asked to run and couldn't be happier that I said yes," she says. "There was a movement to get more women on the ballot across the state, specifically in places where no one was running against an incumbent. Basically, I got sick of complaining and decided to take action. I didn't win, but over 11,000 people voted for me. People are finally waking up to the importance of being engaged in local politics. I will run again. Give me a few years!"

It was a long campaign in which she called on her family and friends to canvass neighborhoods and get out the vote. "My top priorities as a candidate were fully funding our public schools, holding our elected officials accountable, improving traffic, and fighting for affordable housing. It's pretty laughable that I'm considered progressive. I'd say everything I stand for is pretty common sense."

Courtenay walks the walk. She didn't come from fancy roots. She's just a mom, like the rest of us, who is driven to make a better world for her daughter. Courtenay says that after a few years of talking with her friends about creating a place where girls and their moms could talk about important issues and life skills, they decided to go for it, and Girls to the Moon became a reality. "We came up with the name, built a landing page, and grabbed the social media handles all in one night. We started with an event in 2015 and broadened our audience to girls and *all* of their caregivers, not just their moms." Since then they have grown to include an online social network where members can connect and brainstorm with other like-minded girls and caregivers nationwide. The company is for profit. It's still a side gig for all of the founders, but Courtenay's dream is to be full-time COO of the company someday. They believe in empowering their communities while generating profit and supporting other female-owned businesses.

Courtenay's experience of becoming a mom is similar to mine. "Motherhood changed my life," she says. "Having my daughter turned me into a completely different human being. I was a judgmental, angry, and sad woman with very little confidence before I had her, and becoming a mother made me realize I had a lot of room to grow. Raising a productive member of the next generation helped me to become more empathetic, far less judgmental, and a hell of a lot nicer to other people and myself."

Angry, sad, and judgmental are definitely not words I would use to describe her today; confident, determined, and joyful are more like it.

Courtenay's personal and professional choices are impressive, but when I look around the country and talk to people from Baltimore to Little Rock to Los Angeles, I see women just like her in communities from coast to coast. The power is there; the intelligence is there; and the desire to make a difference is clearly there in spades. I suppose I'll catch some hell for generalizing that, as women, we are driven to nurture those around us, but for the most part, that's what I see. Caring about the well-being of others gives us insight and initiative.

Of course, not all of us are prepared to run for office. I know I'm not. But the leadership we need is among us. These women are everywhere, in every city, and we are their megaphones. We must speak loudly and clearly with our voices *and our wallets*—in every neighborhood meeting and every election—about what changes we need to see and the leaders we choose to take us there. And we must show up to vote.

Courtenay looks for holes in the asphalt where people might twist an ankle, and shows up with Redi-Mix to smooth it over. She is doing her part by running for office and starting a company that educates and empowers girls. You can do yours by going to the hospital to hold newborns in detox or volunteering to teach English as a second language or spending an hour a week doing data entry for a domestic violence shelter. Or by spending an hour with a kid you love in a park with no screens in sight. We do our part in our own ways.

Since 1980, an army of women in Mothers Against Drunk Driving reduced drunk driving deaths by 53 percent by advocating for stricter blood alcohol laws nationwide. And an army of women is now working for commonsense gun reform laws through an organization called Moms Demand Action that is striving "to end the epidemic of gun violence that affects every community."[3] These groups are billed as "moms," but they have always included many men, fathers and legislators dedicated to supporting everyone's right to a long, healthy life. This same army of moms (by rite or by nature) is stepping up every day to demand equal pay, equal rights, and equal representation for women because they know it benefits the whole of society.

But to keep hammering away at these changes, we have to keep our energy up.

· · ·

Anyone who has ever experienced the birth of a child or a company or a creative endeavor or political movement; anyone who has ever raised a kid or lost a baby; anyone who has ever lost sleep over something they care passionately about knows the flip side of motherly love. They know the bone-deep fatigue and stress of caring.

If we let it, motherhood can also exhaust us. When we feel undervalued and out of control, and especially when we feel alone, it can make us vulnerable to depression and unhealthy coping mechanisms—which can also make us vulnerable to physical illness. If we are sick or anxiety-ridden, we can't devote the energy we need to the things we want to do.

Caring is hard. The loss of a family member, a pregnancy, a job, a lover, or a pet can derail a person's life for months, if not years, if she doesn't allow herself the time and attention needed to grieve and heal. Even the maddening little annoyances of daily life can take a physical toll on us if we don't heed them. They might seem silly in comparison to big losses, but if they are chronic, they can do real physiological damage.

TAKING CARE

When my son was three years old, we took him to dinner at a Chinese restaurant, hoping against the odds that he might eat tofu and rice like he did when he first started eating solid food. The lobsters in the fish tank captured his attention while we waited for our food, but as soon as it arrived and he saw that dinner did not include a grilled cheese sandwich or French fries, the protesting began. He squirmed and whined about the food set in front of him while his dad and I attempted to enjoy our evening out, and I found myself trumpeting age old maxims like "Don't you know there are kids who would give anything for such a wonderful meal?!" I could feel the stink of anxiety sinking into my gut as we ate. My blood pressure rose, and my stomach turned. The food felt like rocks going down my throat, and I was reminded, viscerally, how our bodies respond to emotional stress.

To be clear, this was a night out for Chinese food in a middle-class American neighborhood with my husband and son, whom I love. There was no real problem. I wasn't sitting there worried about how we would pay for our meal. I wasn't keeping an eye out for suicide bombers. I was just dealing with the standard stress of going out to dinner with a three-year-old at a restaurant, but even so, the impact was palpable.

If that benign situation messed with my stomach, I couldn't help but think about the physical impact on people enduring truly stressful situations: earning minimum wage or less, single parents of sick or disabled kids, refugees, or even teenagers applying to college. Imagine what chronic stress does to *their* digestion and overall health. For all of us, it is incredibly difficult to recognize the physical symptoms of stress in the midst of turmoil—much less address them.

Our job, as caretakers, is to build a society with a support system to reduce and manage these common stressors in every way possible. Not just for kids and for people in dire situations—but for all of us.

We need to hear the distress signals from our own bodies as well as from those around us and have systems in place to ease the pain.

We need daycare. We need rehab. We need food stamps and community gardens. We need decent pay for the folks who care for the elderly and teach our kids. We need a fair tax code. We need clean water and access to health insurance. We need transparent relationships with the police and support for military families. We need protection for women, minorities, immigrants, the disabled, and the LGBTQ community. We need music in the park in the summer and museums and public radio. This stuff shouldn't be controversial. It's about filling basic needs—and the same principles apply for our individual bodies.

We need sustenance, shelter, and clothing. We need freedom of speech in our politics and at home. We need to move our muscles and expand our lungs. We need long walks and a vacation every once in a while. We need dark chocolate, hot tea, and fresh squeezed orange juice. We need friendships, and we need to take care of ourselves while taking care of others.

Our picture of what motherhood is and what it can be is too narrow. Biological motherhood is not a prerequisite for a fully realized, female life. We don't need to bear children in order to love those around us or to advocate for the full potential of civilized society.

I have a feeling that Courtenay would have found her passion for making a difference whether or not she ever had a child. Her passion might not have manifested in exactly the same way, but she would have found it. Her discipline, drive, and desire to serve preceded the fertilized egg nestled in her womb, but when she did become a mom, it informed her. She started making choices that allowed her family and everyone else's families to thrive. Raising a daughter brought her larger purpose into focus.

I used to believe that motherhood would be depleting. Turns out it is, but so is running a campaign, growing a company, going back to school, or anything else that requires your whole self. But motherhood (of any sort) is also inspiring, hilarious, strange, and wonderful.

The most important thing we can do as moms, legislators, and bosses is create safe spaces in every corner of life to let those around us know that they are safe and loved and that we have high expectations of them as stewards of the common good—just like we do for our kids. If we can do that, we will have done everything.

◇◇

Fill in the Fact

I am a mother to _____
_____.

Mothering is life-giving when _____
_____.

Motherhood is exhausting when _____
_____.

Mothering duties I need more help with are _____
_____.

The person/people I am going to ask for that help is/are _____
_____.

Ways I can better care for myself as a mom are _____
_____.

◇◇

Our perspectives need to be at
the forefront of business and
government—not *in spite of* the time
we put in as moms, but *because* of it.

CHAPTER 10

Social Media

Anne Lamott is a San Francisco–based author and outspoken progressive who writes openly about alcoholism, politics, single-motherhood, and the brand of Christianity that welcomes all comers: prostitutes, gays, evangelists, and buttoned-up bankers alike. She is a dreadlocked white lady in her sixties who doesn't mince words or make nice. She has built an astonishing career on her willingness to speak truth about small indignities and the unyielding universal experiences of being alive, particularly as a woman who doesn't color inside the lines.

My dad gave me her book, *Traveling Mercies*, when I was going through a particularly rough patch in my early twenties. He is a minister and a New Testament scholar, so this was not a surprising gift for him to send. I'm sure he held out hope that I would read it and return to my roots, that I would be reminded of the wonderful truth that Christianity can be inclusive and forgiving, a safe place for a wreck like me.

I was never the same after reading that book, but not, perhaps, in the way he hoped. I haven't gone back to the church because it never felt quite like home to me, but Anne's writing taught me that the values of compassion and community I was raised with could transcend my identification with any particular institution. She welcomed me if I wanted to accept the invitation but, also, cut me loose. Her book gave me permission to be a whole, loving, flawed, spiritual, generous, and warm person inside or outside the church. I began to see that I could take those qualities into the world in so many different ways. Being a preacher's kid, that recognition was priceless.

Anne helps her readers feel grounded by letting them know that she is definitely *not* grounded much of the time. If there were an ugly bodily noise that could be made by poetic honesty, she would be making it, loudly, in her writing and probably at the grocery store, too. She sees truth telling as a spiritual practice, and because of her open-armed honesty, millions of her readers are relieved to discover they are not alone. By sharing her truth, she teaches us that it's okay to be a mess, because we're all a mess, and she teaches us how to keep trudging and maintain a sense of humor along the way.

She sets an example for the profoundly healing nature of open communication, and in the modern world, much of the communication we send and receive comes through social media. Anne has made this an art form. She writes long essays on Facebook, giving voice to the ways so many of us feel, and tweets snarky or encouraging messages on Twitter, true to form. In a recent tweet after a brutal health care vote in Congress, she wrote, "I hope the snakes get you. I mean that in a loving, Christian way." She is a master of walking the curved lines that connect two overlapping circles, a Venn diagram of darkness and light. She opens windows into what it's like to move through life in both amazement and horror, windows we know all too well ourselves. She shows up as she is. No pretense, just truth and light.

SOCIAL MEDIA FOR GOOD

At its best, social media has the potential to make us all feel less alone, to make us laugh and ease our minds. To find out how it can best be used this way, I talked to Kate Hays, a digital marketing and social media expert in Washington, DC, who specializes in social enterprise and helping cause-driven organizations get the word out about their work.[1] She was previously vice president of social media and digital outreach at Ogilvy, one of the largest advertising firms in the country and has now started her own company called North & Main.[2]

Kate appreciates a good joke. She's not afraid to be funny. She's also not afraid to be honest, and she knows how to spread good in the world. So I called to ask her about successful online campaigns that have combined darkness and light to produce positive social change.

She said the best example of that in recent years was the "ice bucket challenge" that went viral in 2014. It raised over $220 million for ALS research and led to a breakthrough in treatment a few years later. She told me, "It was started by a bunch of twenty-something guys who wanted to do something funny to raise awareness of ALS after a close friend was diagnosed with it." The original purposes of it were to support their friend, to get some laughs, and to raise some money. The fact that it went viral was a bonus.

ALS is scary. It strikes randomly and destroys the nervous system but leaves the mind intact. There is no cure. Most of us are aware of the disease because of famous people who have suffered from it, such as Lou Gehrig and Steven Hawking. To respond to this terrible disease by pouring a bucket of ice over your head on a hot summer day and posting the video online to raise awareness is bizarre and fun. Challenging your friends to do the same is even more fun, and watching the people you challenged post videos of themselves shrieking and shivering in the following days is flat-out hilarious. It was a flash in the pan, but it raised real money and real awareness. And it made a real difference.

Most of what we do online won't create that kind of explosive impact, but if we approach our social media like they did theirs—with humor, compassion, and playfulness—we can use it to support the well-being of our immediate circles and, hopefully, bigger circles as well with #truthandlight.

The ice bucket challenge brought together that magical combination of darkness and light—Anne Lamott–style. It looked fear in the face and said, *Damn you, Evil Lord of the Underworld! We're going to have a laugh, whether you like it or not.*

When you see something that needs fixing, nag it and tag it on social media.

- Do a black-and-white photo series of homeless people in your neighborhood standing arm in arm with people on their way to work. Put faces and first names to the problem of homelessness.

- Take shots of potholes, and draw funny pictures of city buses, people on skis, and witches on broomsticks crashing into them—and tag the location and the mayor on every one.

- If you're trying to learn to paint, and you're really bad at it but want to get better, take shots of your paintings. Share them online with a request for pointers or a crack about how the bulky body and giant eyes on that dog are totally meant to be an artistic statement about breed discrimination against pit bulls. You'll be amazed by how many people love the work, and maybe a friend will offer to come over and paint with you—or, even better, pose in a bathing suit and an inner tube by a dried up lake bed for your #WheresTheWater series.

TRUTH AND LIGHT ON AND OFFLINE

Exposing ourselves as absurdly, painfully human lightens the weight of bearing it all alone: screaming when the ice water hits, or sharing the frustration of a long commute or the anxiety of studying for exams. If we can capture that spirited vulnerability in our daily feeds (and in our lives at large), we will lessen our own pain and reduce the suffering of people around us, too.

Kate has personally experienced the outpouring of #truthandlight that results when you take a risk and get vulnerable online. She has two healthy little girls, but in the process of trying to conceive them, she and her husband also had two miscarriages. She says, "When I've posted, not even explicitly, but when I've hinted that we've lost two pregnancies—that this happened to us and it happens to people all the time—those posts always get the most attention because there is something real and genuine about them." Miscarriages are awful and common. They occur in 10–20 percent of pregnancies.[3] Everyone hurts for a loss like that whether they have experienced it themselves or not, so when a friend or stranger is willing to come out and say, *It happened. I survived, and you are not alone,* people respond because they can connect.

Truth on social media can offer hope in tragedy. It can also offer solace for a plethora of quiet insecurities that plague our daily lives, the ones that hover in our minds but go unspoken.

• • •

Before Instagram was ever a thing, Anne Lamott gave me the gifts of liberty and perspective through a few sentences in *Traveling Mercies*. I read that book in the years before social media became what it is today. In it, she writes, "Even though I am a feminist and even though I am religious, I secretly believe in some mean little rat part of my brain, that I *am* my skin, my hair, and worst of all, those little triangles that pooch at the top of my thighs. In other words, that I am my packaging."[4]

When I first read that passage, I thought, *The triangles! Oh my God, I hate my triangles, too!* And I was no longer alone. Not only that, but in her serene but subversive way, Anne reminded me that I was more than my packaging. Clearly she was more than *her* packaging. She was smart and wise and irreverent, and I wanted to be just like that. So if her triangles didn't define her in my eyes, mine shouldn't define me either.

The triangles may seem like a silly thing, but if I'm being honest, they are the #1 genetic characteristic that I would change about my body if I could. Even more than my fragile knees or weak vision, the triangles would have to go. Every day from puberty until just a couple of years ago, when I put on my clothes and stared in the mirror, I thought about how awful the triangles were, how wide they made me look, and what I could do to disguise or change them. Even now, those thoughts arise sometimes. But Anne made my fixation funny and a little bit ridiculous.

So a few years later, when I stood up in front of a room full of students at Vanderbilt University to talk about body image and eating disorders, I was able to step out from behind the podium to point out my triangles and to talk about how they fueled my own eating disorder when I was in college. By stepping out and speaking up, I showed how much bigger they were in my own mind than they were in reality and exposed the irrational absurdity of starving ourselves and picking our bodies to pieces. The whole room laughed, at my expense— including me—and after that, the triangles weren't so bad anymore. They became a visual reminder of liberty, of how close I am to not giving a damn anymore. Yes, they're pointy, and they're mine.

The power Anne claimed on those paper pages is no different than the power she claims online today, but these days, you don't need a book deal or a podium at a college to reach large numbers of people. All of us can step out and speak up any time we want.

Social media is pervasive. We are glued to imagery all day, every day, via the devices in our pockets, which is often seen as a detriment to our well-being—but it also means the capability is in our hands to mold and shape that imagery. It's in our kids' hands as well, and if used properly, social media can be a formidable force for positive change. We can upend the ways women and their bodies are perceived by hoisting new images up onto pedestals and freeing ourselves from the unrealistic imagery that has dogged us since the dawn of digital media. We have the opportunity to visually redefine what beauty and strength look like for the next generation, both digitally and in real life.

Body positive advertising campaigns have multiplied rapidly in recent years. Dove's ImageHack.org campaign flooded a well-known stock photography site with photographs of "strong, independent and original women in non-stereotypical settings" and tagged the photos with phrases like "beautiful woman" or "strong woman."[5] The campaign launched in Denmark, and the images were picked up by advertisers and agencies all over the country. It's progress, but if you Google "beautiful woman," the search images still yield almost exclusively photos of very thin, white women in contorted positions with peekaboo shoulders, generous cleavage, and long, lanky legs. We are making a dent, but there is still a giant metal wall standing infuriatingly erect in our way.

My monthly newsletter takes a page from Dove's playbook. I share images tagged as #StrengthOutsideIn, pictures of brave people trying new things, laughing unconsciously, strengthening their bodies, and reveling in living. It's my little contribution. It's small, but it matters to me and my readers. People reach out all the time to say, *I never thought of beauty that way before. Thank you for highlighting these people!* We can all do the same for our personal networks. If we flood the internet with these images, we can begin to shame and crowd out the flimsy, uninteresting portrayals of beauty we see so often online.

Call out beauty when you see it in your friends and in strangers. Post those images so we can see through your eyes what beauty looks like—all sizes, all races, all different levels of ability and accomplishment. It's your circle of influence. Use it for #physicaldisobedience, for #truthandlight.

External portrayals of beauty make a difference in the ways we see ourselves. When we see celebrities like America Ferrera posting photos of herself training for a half-marathon, tired but joyful and proud of her accomplishments and her body, we are both reassured and inspired. But it's important to incorporate that appreciation into our real lives as well, beyond the virtual world and into the physical one, so we not only see beauty differently but *perceive* it differently in our bodies and respond accordingly when we witness a betrayal of it.

We can speak the truth. We can hashtag *#beauty* in authentic ways. We can tweet about how a three-mile run turned into a peaceful, two-mile stroll, and Instagram about how fantastic it is to feel sweat pouring down our backs, purging toxic, political bullshit from our crystal clear veins. We can glorify the beauty and effort we see in our friends and family members, even (and especially) when they can't appreciate it themselves. But if we post about how sexy natural beauty is and then refuse to go out in public without "perfect" hair and makeup, we fail. If we post about strong, capable thighs and then spend hours online researching liposuction, we are not being honest. I have been that person. I have posted that "this is the year I start wearing shorts again" in praise of my legs just as they are—before making an appointment to have my triangles marked up by a middle-aged man with plastic cheekbones and a Sharpie.

I didn't follow through, of course. The triangles are holding strong.

Putting on a front isolates us in secrecy. It turns us into paper doll versions of ourselves, frail and liable to blow away at the slightest hint of wind. We love our friends for their honesty when they are brave enough to share. If we hope to bend the influence of social media toward the light, we need a collective agreement to bear witness to the truth—our own truth and the truth we see in the world—and we need to do it with a certain je ne sais quoi, a deafening whoopee cushion of pro-body self-love.

TAKING IT INTO THE REAL WORLD

The same principles apply when we look beyond our bodies, into the broader world, at the issues of human rights we hope to influence.

"If you're someone who flippantly throws out a #BlackLivesMatter tweet," Kate says, "but then you don't stand up for the woman in your grocery store line who isn't getting respect from the cashier, then that's not really doing much to change the world. By posting, you can feel like you're off the hook for doing something real, in person, face-to-face, but we're not off the hook for that. So we need to ask, 'what does it look like to be consistent online and offline?'"

This is called hashtag activism. You get the social cred for being part of the movement without actually showing up to a meeting with the police chief about body cameras. We've all been guilty of it at one time or another, usually because we're stretched too thin to begin with. We want to contribute but have to be at work from 8 to 6; the kids need help with their homework at night; and on the weekend, we can't make it to three different rallies while running all over town to pick up prescriptions and restock the fridge. If we're lucky, we might get an hour with a friend and a bottle of wine to process the insanity of the week.

Posting and hashtagging does make some difference. It shapes the public conversation.

Calling your congressperson is even better. It lets the people who make the laws know where their constituents stand and that we are watching.

Showing up in person to help in your city matters most of all. It builds bridges that never existed before, and that means somebody is going to make it to the polls who never voted before and a kid is going to have a warm jacket who never had one before. Community connections and interactions are also notorious for easing symptoms of depression. They reduce feelings of isolation and renew our faith in humanity.

Doing good isn't just a charitable act; it's also a wonderful way to take better care of yourself.

But even after all of that outreach, sometimes it doesn't seem like enough when we lay our heads down on the pillow at night. It's rewarding to see small victories come to fruition, but keeping our energy up can still be exhausting. We are working to shed light on the darkness, but, in the meantime, too often, we forget to lighten up. We forget to make our activism fun.

ART, MONEY, AND GETTING OUT THE VOTE

Every town in every county has musicians, artists, poets, and writers who are throwing light on the truth in ways that make us laugh and cry in spite of ourselves. They make the slog palatable. This has always been true, but sometimes we neglect to acknowledge those voices. Spirituals rose out of American slavery. Visual art has reflected native cultures over centuries. Graffiti and rap gave voice to urban life in the 1980s when *no one* was listening to those communities. And the protest music of the 1960s cut an entire generation loose.

When I look around at the campaigns that are thriving in my own community in spite of the activist fatigue that so many of us are experiencing—the ones getting press with crowds lining up around the corner—they all have one thing in common. They are intertwined with local artists who are reflecting the times. In addition to raising money or awareness, they are also offering relief: visual art, music, film, theater, and dance. They are providing an outlet for those of us in the daily grind to whistle while we work.

It seems like people at the highest levels of policy sometimes forget to let the message breathe. They want to cram into our ears all the words they can manage about injustice and the next steps for involvement. But there are too many words and too many plans to sustain. Artists, on the other hand, can hold us in the palm of their hands with a melody and a mission to #keepgoing. They can also normalize left-leaning voices in conservative pockets of the country to make it known that it's okay to think differently and to be proud of progressive political beliefs.

We forget, from time to time, that posting fifteen outraged

articles a day on Facebook disappears into a wash of political dismay. But posting a painting of a women with sunken eyes sitting bolt upright in defiance says more than the pundits ever could.

In Nashville, my hometown, we have an embarrassment of riches in this department. Some of the most beloved performers in town are writing cathartic, compelling songs like "White Man's World" by Jason Isbell, "When They Go Low We Go High" by Ruby Amanfu, "Stronger Together" by Mary Gauthier, "Same Blood" by Kyshona Armstrong, "Thoughts and Prayers" by Will Hoge, "Remember Love Wins" by Nicki Bluhm, and "Pay Gap" by Margo Price.

Sally Jaye and her partner Brian Wright have a small, independent record label called Café Rooster Records, built on the simple principle that it's possible to cut out the middleman and funnel a lot more money back to the artists.[6] They put out a compilation record in 2017 entitled *Strange Freedom: Songs of Love and Protest*, featuring songs like "Mercy Now" by Mary Gauthier and "All That I Require" by Radney Foster. One-hundred percent of the proceeds from that record go to Planned Parenthood.

Stacie Huckeba is a well-known music photographer who lives just down the road. She has photographed icons such as Dolly Parton and Buddy Guy as well as rising stars such as Aaron Lee Tasjan and Elizabeth Cook. Her recent exhibit, called "This Shoe Doesn't Fit," featured an eclectic array of photos taken of people of every stripe—men, women, and children of every race and socioeconomic class—wearing a size 7 pair of golden, rhinestone-studded, high-heeled Ivanka Trump shoes.[7] Her profits from that series go to Planned Parenthood as well.

The local fashion industry has exploded in recent years with designers such as Amanda Valentine, Manuel, and Imogene + Willie growing at breakneck speed and desperately in need of a highly-skilled workforce. So the Nashville Fashion Alliance partnered with Catholic Charities to train refugees, primarily from Africa and Asia, for long-term job placements at the Omega Apparel Factory, an old military uniform factory that was in danger of shutting down. More jobs plus more support for refugee communities plus more fashion equals a huge win for the city.

This movement is not unique to Nashville. We are just a little blue dot in the middle of one of the reddest states in the nation. You can bet—if this quality of art and innovation is coming out of here—it is being matched in Portland and Atlanta and Milwaukee. Every city does not have the resources of Los Angeles, Chicago, New York, or Nashville, but they all have beloved bands and local artists with diverse fan bases that can bring out a crowd. We need those crowds now. We need them to register to vote and come out to the polls. To get them to do this, instead of reaching out solely online, we need to show them a good time in real life.

Let's bring together music, visual art, fundraising, and voter registration drives leading up to every election.

Let's plaster the country with free music festivals, featuring our favorite bands and arts and crafts booths. Artists can sign on to be part of a nationwide network with a mission to drive voter registration and pledge 10 percent of their merch profits from the events to Emerge America, Headcount, Indivisible, or Planned Parenthood.

The only requirement for entry? They have to listen to their favorite artists nagging them all day to visit the voter registration booth next to the beer tent. And text three friends to remind them to register as well.

The artists get exposure; the causes get cold, hard cash; and the voter rolls get boosted by tens of thousands of people who need a reason to show up.

I ran this idea past Rebecca Davis, a digital strategist and founder and CEO of Ovington, a consulting firm that works to build capacity and expand the reach of nonprofits and groups like the American Association for the Advancement of Science. Rebecca worked to support the DC chapter of the Women's March and is heavily involved with galvanizing sanctuary churches to accompany immigrants to routine ICE check-in meetings to make sure they are able to come back home to their families.

"There is so much disillusionment," she said, "but events like what you're describing have a fighting chance of bringing in broader-based groups because they don't have the hang ups of the political parties. It's a compelling balance of reality and celebration. The name of the game is getting a group of influential folks who can speak to their own audiences about what you're trying to do. The authenticity and honesty of that connection is cathartic, both for the individuals who are doing the storytelling or making the art as well as for the people out there who can relate to them."

We don't have to be geniuses to realize that we might get a few more people to fill out a registration form if we draw them in with a song or a ceramic vase. This can happen at every level, from grass-roots to massive organizations. Artists don't have to be international superstars to hold sway with their email lists, and these messages can come together in our own twitter feeds as well. We'll get a whole lot further with some tunes in the background, especially if we're also spreading the word about artists we love who are promoting causes we can get behind.

• • •

There is poetry in the dance between darkness and light. There is something enticing there, but we can't discover that poetry if our minds are consumed with dogma and rage half the time and with appearing perfect the other half. We allow so little time for daydreaming. The newsfeed scrolls down the page, and we are increasingly frozen, overcome by the sheer number of people being profiled, incarcerated, defunded, lied to, or belittled.

We need to keep showing up as often as we can, and the whole thing will be a lot less painful with music and beer on tap.

Let's make the most of it, online and off. It's up to us to dump an ice bucket on our social media feeds every once in awhile, and it's up to us to drag our guitar-playing friends out onto street corners across the country for grassroots voter registration drives and to call for the larger organizations we support to think outside the box.

We're dealing with heavy issues. Lives truly are at stake, but a little bit of nonsense goes a long way toward keeping our spirits up and inviting fresh eyes and ears into the fold to set the movement alight.

I know you're tired
And you ain't sleeping well
Uninspired
And likely mad as hell
But wherever you are
I hope the high road leads you home again
To a world you want to live in.

—Jason Isbell[8]

✕✕

Fill in the Fact

I am using my social media feed for both truth and light
(circle one):   True   False

Inspiring voices in my social media feed are _____
_____.

Ways I can support those voices are _____
_____.

Ways I can reflect those voices in my real life are _____
_____.

Discouraging themes in my feed are _____
_____.

Ways I can reduce exposure to those themes are _____
_____.

I can promote this event/fund-raiser on social media _____
_____.

I will make it fun by _____
_____.

◇◇

Call out beauty when you see
it in your friends and strangers.
It's your circle of influence. Use
it for #physicaldisobedience
and #truthandlight.

CHAPTER 11

Rest

In the words of indie rock darlings, the Dead Horses:

> *Sometimes I wish I was a leaf.*
> *Sometimes I wish I was a tall tree.*
> *Sometimes I wish I was a deep sea swimmer.*
>
> *Sometimes I wish I was a rock.*
> *Sometimes I wish I was a tall corn stalk.*
> *Sometimes I wish to be anything I'm not.*[1]

Sometimes I wish to make all the noise stop. Every last bit of me wants to shut down and dig a hole in my covers. Or hit the road.

Sometimes it seems impossible to hit pause—but sometimes I get my priorities straight. I remember I'm no good to anybody if I can't move my arm or if I'm so exhausted that I'm half-witted and driving up on curbs.

Sometimes the most valuable thing I can do for my work, friends, family, and the world is to stop all the things I'm supposed to do. And do new things instead. Or no things at all. And be alive for a bit, just for the hell of it.

Our muscles need time to heal between workouts to grow stronger, and our minds need time away from the incessant drive to achieve to home in on what will bring our plans to fruition.

When you are forever wrapped up in conquering all the things, you are a servant to the minutia of your life. So yes, physical disobedience is about pushing your body to get stronger and eat real food and wear clothes that empower you, but it's also about saying: *Nope. This has to stop. I need a minute.*

We are masters of reaching out to help others in need. When neighbors are going through times of crisis, we start meal calendars to make sure they're fed. When friends have babies, we pop in to take over for a few hours so the parents can run errands or take a nap. At home, we take on the cerebral task of organizing endless appointments, bill payments, household labor splits, and schedule coordination. We do all of this by choice. It feels good to get things done, but too often, we forget (or simply decline) to *step away* when we desperately need the relief.

Too many things. We can't do this forever. We *shouldn't* do it forever.

Everybody needs something from you. Drop off, pick up, meeting, fund-raiser, planning committee, work out, set the clock, here we go. But what about aimlessness? What about being a living creature for a minute instead of a hero.

"Rest" is about more than just sleep. It's also about play. It's about prying your mind loose from your routine, seeing a new place, talking with a new person, trying a new activity, or giving yourself the grace to close your eyes and be still.

Inspiration, the kind everyone is scrambling so hard to achieve, resides in downtime. If you don't take time off, you won't get anywhere near inspired. You will stall and possibly even collapse.

We should all have the chance to sit on a porch in a comfortable chair, with just the right amount of sun, just the right amount of shade, and not a care in the world. But not everybody gets that time.

Rest is a luxury. There is no doubt about that. We can't all manage to take a day at a spa or on a mountaintop, or even a few hours off from work, but we *can* all step away for at least a few minutes to take a deep breath with our faces turned to the sun. We can put on our headphones and play a song that lifts us up. We can stop checking things off the list and call a friend. We can sit down on a swing in an empty playground or take a bus to the outskirts of town where buildings and pavement make way for dirt roads and giant magnolia trees. Leaning in isn't always the answer. Sometimes we need to lean out and let the force of the wind hold us up.

Work and relationships are at the center of everything we love. They are important. The people and things that matter to us deserve us at our best, but we can't be at our best if we're beat to hell and stymied by fatigue.

My clients drive me nuts with this destructive desire to keep going when it's obvious they need a break. When they're fixated on a new workout plan or dealing with a promotion or job loss, birth, death, divorce, move, major project, or any other monumental effort or change, it is nearly impossible to get them to slow down. There are a million things that need to be done. Motivation is high—frantic even—and the road ahead is long. But when that hectic energy kicks in, it howls to be cut loose so it can fly up into the far reaches of consciousness and return with fresh solutions.

Buckling down doesn't always yield the results we want. Every commitment we care about suffers if we don't take time to linger. But when we stop striving to be anything other than what we are, where we are, we make time and space for inspiration to strike. So bugger off. Give yourself a minute of nothing at all.

CREATIVITY AND COSTUMES

Intellectual exploration requires time and space, and nobody knows more about that than the teachers who work in our schools every day to engage kids, of all ages, in learning.

Julia Hoge is an elementary school counselor who utilizes cutting-edge, evidence-based research about how kids' minds develop and expand. She told me, "No child grows more or learns more than when they just play with one another. Kids need movement and someone to catalyze engagement in activities like learning games, cheers, reading in costume (or in a laundry basket or a tree house), and lots of breaks to play. Play boosts problem-solving ability, emotional regulation, language development, personal awareness, and more."

When kids sit around staring at a chalkboard with their legs chained to their desks, their brains shut down. When they connect with their bodies and give their minds space to soar, they reengage and come to class ready to learn. Julia said, "Research shows that if kids ages five to ten get just five minutes of meditation a day, their sleep improves, relationships improve, and overall happiness goes up."

So, yeah. Schools are starting to apply this knowledge in their classrooms. Those of us who are parents are lobbying administrators for more recess, more art, more physical education. It's great for kids, but what about us? The need for physical activity and a break from the norm is no different for adults. We don't grow up and suddenly stop needing to play and sleep and dream. Our creativity is squashed by the same old schedule, the drone of the twenty-four-hour news cycle, and the stimulation of screens and more screens. We are consumed by deadlines and dieting apps, forever chasing external metrics and reminding ourselves that we are falling short.

Paraphrasing Rumi, Julia said, "We are looking in the branches for what is actually at the root." We desperately want to improve our focus. *What did I come in here to do? Where is that file? Why isn't anyone calling me back?!* But if you're legitimately burned out, buckling down doesn't necessarily help. Your project might be much better served by going to the root, animating your body and brain in ways that have nothing to do with the work itself. If you're feeling beat, a jog or a nap, a change of venue or outfit, can go a long way toward helping you find that lost file and zeroing in on the work at hand.

When you move, oxygen-rich blood pumps through your brain and neurotransmitters come to life, activating learning, memory, and overall cognition. When you awaken from your nap, you'll be more alert and creative and much less likely to leave your coffee on the roof of your car. When you travel to a new place, you nurture a sense of independence and force your mind to adapt to new circumstances. And when you're comfortable in your clothes on a lunch date, your body language is warmer, more open, and you're much more likely to connect.

While you're busy doing all of that, you'll forget about the folks not calling you back, and the lost file will wondrously appear in the magazine rack next to the toilet.

Thus, inspired by Julia and her merry band of first graders, as I write this, I am sporting a hot pink wig and a trucker hat, and—wouldn't you know it—the words come easier this way.

Whether writing a book, dreaming up a design for a new website, organizing an event, or trying to coordinate the schedules of five family members running in different directions, we would all do well to set the work aside sometimes. We can learn a lot from Julia and people like her: nurses, teachers, and social workers—people working in helping professions—who are saving lives every day, guiding kids and their families through crises and into healthier life choices. We desperately need their creativity and insight, and in order for them to offer their skills effectively, they need to give themselves a break as well. They need decent pay and vacations. They need enough people on staff that they don't have to be on-call six out of seven nights a week. They need a breather, and so do the rest of us.

Julia adores her job ensuring that students have what they need to do their best in school, but it's no small task to stay centered while witnessing (and having to intervene in) issues such as child abuse and neglect. So Julia incorporates the lessons she teaches her students in her own life as well.

"Practices of self-care and personal grace are critical," she said. "I incorporate mindfulness and/or yoga daily. Even if it's been a great day, taking some time in the quiet is the only way to survive. I reenergize when I read; when I'm around my brilliant friends that challenge me; when I connect with myself and my family; when I laugh; when I don't do the dishes; when I throw out things I don't need. Being where my feet are builds me up to be ready for my life that I love."

MAKING AIMLESSNESS ACCESSIBLE

Almost everyone I asked about their rituals of rest and play indicated that they don't even think about decompressing often enough—and following through to take time out is even harder—but our bodies disintegrate under fire. The drumbeat of bills to pay, calendars to sync, relationships to sustain, friendships to support, children to care for, cars to fix, meetings to attend, campaigns to champion, homes to clean, and meals to cook can drive a person crazy.

We need to drift and remind each other how much rest matters. We need to grab our friends by the sleeve and say: You're coming with me. Folding chairs in the yard.

If we don't kick back, we will shrivel into shells of our former selves. This stuff directly impacts our health. Being exhausted makes us impulsive. It triggers cravings and makes healthy decisions infinitely harder to carry out. It leaves us frustrated, lethargic, and guilty that we aren't able to self-motivate. But we can't burn energy we don't have. We have to renew it somehow, and we can't do that by hammering on a bent nail. Time away is the explosive ingredient that allows us to get the job done and done well.

The inability to step away from daily responsibilities is one of many reasons why poverty is so incredibly unfair. If you're working multiple jobs for the basic survival of yourself and your family, there isn't space for daydreaming. There isn't time for innovative, abstract thought, or for meal planning for that matter. Of course people in poverty tend to have higher obesity rates and eat fast food more frequently. Fast food is a quick and easy source of pleasure, and we all need and deserve pleasure. If I had three kids and three jobs, I'd be tempted to grab French fries and a shake for dinner at the end of the day, too—quick, inexpensive, tasty calories, an easy choice.

Brand-new parents have a similar dilemma. Tired and strung out, they try to reclaim their "me-time" in unhealthy ways after work or after the kids go to sleep. They feel like their lives are not their own, that their days are possessed by everyone else's demands, so they go on the defensive. *I'm staying awake to watch another episode, damn it, because this is my time, and I'm going to have another drink and a bag of chips, too, because I deserve it! I deserve to stay up and eat what I want and enjoy myself on my own terms.* But stuffing ourselves before bed or staying up late when we're already drained aren't acts of self-preservation. They are acts of self-destruction.

This is why paid vacation, paid family leave, and access to affordable health care are so important. Those programs allow us to breathe. With those safeguards in place, if we allow ourselves, we can put our feet up, undisturbed, to be alive and okay for a little while every day.

CHOOSING TO STOP

Because of the United States' lack of those support systems, I thought Americans might be alone in this dilemma. We have a reputation for being overly ambitious and working too much—but surprisingly, when I spoke to women from all over the world, I found that the tendency to work beyond capacity seems all too common. The impulse to overcommit appears to be a nearly universal Achilles heel for women. We care a lot and work too much, but when we're able to step out of that rhythm, *everyone* benefits.

The CFO of a major art museum in Cape Town, South Africa, told me that for her, "Stress manifests physically. If I don't remember to stop, my body tells me that I have to. The first sign is migraines and the second is 'I just can't get out of bed today.' By then, it's too late. If I focus on work output only, over time, it definitely results in less creative, less productive, generally pedestrian work. I can't give output if I don't also find a way of refilling myself." She said that working too hard and paying too little attention to her personal needs is her "default stage."

In recent years, she has made a conscious effort to change that. She negotiated thirty days of paid vacation in her current job. When she's not working, she goes mountain biking, reads, immerses herself in theater and art, and goes dancing with friends. And once a year, she steps away completely with no cell phone service for four days in the African desert at an event called AfrikaBurn, South Africa's official Burning Man event. It's a temporary city that springs up out of the desert on empty land that is transformed once a year by an all-volunteer staff into a cauldron of art installations, sculpture, costumes, music, and "mutant vehicles"—a retreat from regular life dedicated to nurturing the creativity of all who want to come.

"There is no other place I could go that gives me the same sense of play as an adult," she said. "I get to spend four days in the desert with my mates. Nothing could replace it."

Another woman, a Canadian who abandoned a lucrative career as a brand manager for a global cosmetic company in Toronto, told me, "I devoted my life to the job, and everything else fell by the wayside: my health, my marriage, my friendships, and social life. I had a pretty big meltdown. It was spurred by work stress mostly. When my marriage imploded, it led to a series of events where I pulled a giant 360 on my life—for the better. I went from a high-pressured, high-stress, chaotic life to a much simpler one."

She teaches creativity and innovation to college students in Switzerland now. When they are stuck, she tells them to "seek out different stimulus and raw materials, different experiences or activities; pick up a new magazine or newspaper; talk to someone you wouldn't normally chat with; travel, etc. It fills their kaleidoscopes with bits and bobs that get combined in a myriad of different ways to produce ideas for work, family, and life. I find their perspectives so uplifting, untarnished, and full of hope. It has a positive ripple effect in all aspects of my life."

We forget to appreciate the potential of curiosity, raw physicality, silence and sound, and a lack of any agenda—but every one of those practices pays off generously.

• • •

Outside the windows of my gym, where my clients come to exercise each day, there are squirrels, rabbits, opossums, lizards, wild hare, and a menagerie of birds. They jump, hop, slither, crawl, and fly all day long while we jump, hop, slither, and crawl on the other side of the glass. We would fly, too, if we could.

I don't live in a rural area. I'm in a densely populated neighborhood directly adjacent to the heart of a major metropolitan city, but the world somehow sustains this incredible array of wildlife in the middle of vast concrete and urban sprawl. Because if this, every day, I am reassured that the natural world is strong. It surges and thrives where, by all rights, it should falter and fail.

Humans have that same natural tendency to thrive, but we have a blind spot that will crush us if we don't take heed. We are not taking the time needed to replenish our reserves. But if we allow ourselves to indulge a little—in wigs and trucker hats, museums and mountains, recipes and roller coasters—we will flourish as well.

We know what we want. We're doing the legwork. We have the expertise to achieve it, but *OH MY GOD, WHY THE HELL HASN'T IT HAPPENED YET, AND WHAT CAN I DO TO MAKE IT BUDGE? I'm supposed to be fifteen pounds lighter by now. I should be making more money. I was supposed to have a baby by the time I was thirty-five. My dream should be taking off faster than this. I wanted to cure cancer by now, damn it. I need to work harder, faster, with more dedication. I'm not doing enough!*
GASP.GURGLE.CHOKE.

We are attempting to bend the universe to our will. We impose this tyranny on our bodies, relationships, careers, and all of the problems we hope to fix. We force it on the passing minutes of our lives until the minutes surrender and slip away. It's nuts. When we strangle our lives this way, we injure our bodies and sabotage our goals.

So here's the deal:

If it is 9 a.m. on a rainy Saturday morning and your kid was up all night with a fever while thunder and lightning pounded you—stay cloistered together in bed, buried in a mound of covers with a pile of books.

If it's Friday night and people at work are pressuring you to go out for drinks but you want to go home and be with your fur baby—wave good-bye, put a leash on the puppy, and take a stroll in the dark.

If it is midday on Tuesday and the news is bad, your phone has been ringing all morning, and you don't have words left to speak—leave the vibration on your desk, crawl into the driver's seat of your car with the window cracked and the engine off, lean your seat as far back as it will go, and close your eyes to unwind in silence.

If it is Monday morning and you just had the most wonderful weekend of your life, you said "I do" to the most beautiful person you have ever known and danced until dawn with all of the people you love, you made brunch and dinner for the diehards that remained the following day and lay entwined with your lover all night—get up with coffee, moving slow.

And if it is the dead of August and you've been slaving like a pack mule at work for the last eight months with no vacation in sight—ask your boss for a long weekend and tell her that you'll be a better, more productive human when you return. Get in your car or hitch a ride on a bus, plane, or train bound for the mountains or the beach; bring a book, sneakers, and flip-flops; and remove yourself entirely from everything you're "supposed to do." Bring a friend if you want, but ditch the kids if possible.

Rest. In the name of everything you care about, give yourself time whenever you can.

• • •

There is no accomplishment that has to be achieved by the time you're thirty years old. Or forty. Or fifty. It's a long road to the next degree or the next job or the family you hope to have someday, but if you let it, in the meantime, life will keep expanding and quivering as you go. Simple pleasures are right in front of you. Liberty can happen here and now, but you have to make time for it. Nobody else is going to give it to you. This is a gift you have to give to yourself.

Step outside. Take off your shoes, and stand in the grass. Eat a rice crispy treat and stare at the moon. Please. You will be so much happier and more powerful for having done so.

◇◇

Fill in the Fact

The last time I took a personal day was _____

_____.

The last time I took a trip with friends was _____

_____.

The next personal day or trip I will take is _____

_____.

One way I can take a few minutes for myself every day is _____

_____.

I can get a little more sleep at night by _____

_____.

Once a month I will check out a new (circle one):

Film   Exhibit   Club   Sport   Concert   Class   Book

Next month, specifically, _____

_____.

When I go to this new place, _____, I will
(circle one):

Take my friend/partner _____ with me.

Go by myself.

◇◇

Be alive for a bit, just
for the hell of it.

PART 3

MIND UNGLUED

CHAPTER 12

Turning Points

I am sitting on the beach, wearing a bikini I bought last year to show off my only tattoo, one I got in tribute to my son and all of the creatures (human or otherwise) that I wish I could put in my pocket and protect forever.

Sitting here alone, I look out at the ocean and sink into what it's like to bask in my body the way it is, in my muscles, skin, wrinkles, and fleshy tummy. I think about years past when I struggled over what bathing suit to wear; how much to cover up as I walked along the water; how to avoid sitting in the sand with stomach rolls showing; or which foods might make me bloat like a puffer fish. I lie back on my towel, splayed out, feeling the sand on my hands and feet, shells in my fingers, and grit between my toes. My body releases into the ground, and the mushy parts flatten out so the birds and clouds can see my wideness. *What the hell was I thinking to never lie back like this before?*

The old pose comes to mind, and I try it. Knees bent just so. A little arch in my low back. Shoulders down. Chest out. *Oh yes, super comfortable and totally relaxing.* And I start to laugh out loud, alone on a beach towel, digging my toes deeper into the sand, flipping them up and digging some more. The laugh settles into a chuckle and then a catch in my throat.

There is nowhere more elemental than the beach, nowhere it makes less sense to be body conscious. All the summers I spent sitting around thinking about my butt and thighs—what a waste, what a huge ridiculous fail.

There is nothing I can do to salvage those summers, but, starting now, I can make a practice of catching myself in that bizarre mannequin-twisting. I can neutralize the situation physically and let my body sink into an even stance, peripheral muscles engaging and releasing as intended. When my mind goes to: *Stomach blubber showing. Sit up straight, dumbass.* I can choose instead: *Check out that sandpiper! Where's the Zima?*

• • •

We can't be grounded in the world if we aren't grounded in our bodies. It's really as simple as that.

We can't command respect anywhere, personally or professionally, if we don't respect ourselves, and that includes the state of our bodies. It's impossible to enjoy anything while hating your own flesh, so how do you change those patterns? How do you guide your mind away from defeating thoughts to better appreciate what your body can do?

It starts by forgetting all the diets and schemes and, instead, doing whatever needs to be done to *take care* of yourself so you can genuinely, physically feel better. Once you're doing all you can to nurture your well-being, it's a practice of yielding to a mystical, magical, previously undiscovered carelessness. Find out what it's like to be a person with a body doing bodily things—standing, walking, sitting, seeing, touching, tasting, smelling, hearing, digesting, breathing, and beating. And if you catch yourself wasting brain power again on terrible body image, plant both feet on the ground and take space. Open your arms as wide as you can; roll your shoulders back in broad circles; or wiggle like a sound wave moving through air. Jump up and down until you are standing again, like a legitimate person—a body doing worthwhile things.

Let go of the flawless ghost lady in your mind. Let her float up into the heavens where she and her compatriots can gather poolside at the Sky Bar with skinny margaritas, celery, and energy drinks to keep them going. Fly away, ladies. Be free.

Diet mind-set is keeping us meekly in place. It is bestowing us with the broken belief that we are only as valuable as our measurements. If we want to move on to a balanced, sane society, we have to let it go once and for all. Good health, kindness, smarts, honesty, courage, and love of life are worth idolizing, not big tits and tiny waists. But I can't just sound the trumpets from here behind my keyboard, make a decree, and have it be so.

The cultural turning point we would like to see starts with each one of us recognizing and reconsidering the intimate ways we perceive and interact with our own bodies.

Are you comfortable in a room by yourself naked? It starts by standing upright in your skin—not defiant or ashamed—just mortal, naked, and okay. Once you feel comfortable with that, you can put on clothes that make you feel irresistible and try standing upright in the wider world, expansive and unashamed of your physical self.

From there, you can design and draft and build. You can speak your mind and listen well. You can reach and bend. You can go on a date and eat what you want and sit and move with ease.

I've been toying with this game of physical adaptation in various scenarios lately. I've been curious to find out what happens to a meeting or a shopping trip or exercise class if I'm not constricting my body to fit. It's both disconcerting and remarkably painless. The more ease I experience *being* at the beach, *being* at dinner, *being* at a reunion, the weirder and more unacceptable the old hang-ups seem to be. When I'm not standing awkwardly, my body aligns and tough situations are easier to manage. When I am present and unaffected, distorting the natural stance of my body strikes me as comical, and I am almost unrecognizable to myself.

It takes time and conscious effort to notice the contortions we adopt and replace them with solid footing, but it is well worth the effort.

The choice to be in our bodies without shame is the most important thing each of us can do to facilitate being feminists, caretakers, geeks, revolutionaries, tree huggers, experts, or advocates. We have been living in spite of our bodies when we should have been living through them.

DARE TO DO SOMETHING DIFFERENT

This shift toward dynamic action starts in your body and spreads like lava—a thick layer of authenticity burning its way to larger turning points in your life, moments when you're deciding who you want to be. It's clear when these moments arrive. You know them in your gut. You're faced with a major decision or nagging awareness that something isn't right. You're acutely aware of the desire to go back to school or off birth control, to stay in the city or move back home. You're torn over whether to quit a miserable job or keep working to save up for a trip around the world. These are identity decisions. They're not about who you thought you were or who you're supposed be; they're about who you plan to be from here on out. The choice between old and new stares you in the face and dares you to blink. It becomes painfully clear that you have no option but to *do something* about the dissonance, or lose a little bit of yourself. The "not rightness" of avoiding the decision seeps into every other aspect of your life, and you have to make a move because not doing so would mean giving up on yourself.

This is the moment to turn back to your physical health for reinforcement. When you're caught in the vortex of indecision and can't think straight, try any or all of these:

- Get up in the morning, and start your day with fifteen minutes of walking or jogging or stretching or biking or yoga or meditation or dancing or boxing or singing.

- Eat breakfast.
- Pack snacks.
- Climb a hill.
- Climb a wall.
- Jump rope.
- Swim.
- Learn to juggle.
- Learn to knit.
- Take a public-speaking class.
- Call a friend to kvetch and stretch.
- Plank.
- Hula-hoop.
- Do a handstand against the wall, or if you can't do that, lie down with your legs straight up the wall.
- Visit a park or mountain or beach you've never visited before.
- Lie in bed and kick and scream and lose your shit. Full-on temper tantrum. It's highly therapeutic.
- Keep doing all of these things, and anything else you can think of to get your body moving in new directions, until you figure out what to do next.

Changing the position or velocity of your body literally opens your mind. No matter how in or out of shape you might be, doing something that strengthens you will ground you in the truth and give you the clarity of mind necessary to ask for a raise, leave the douchebag in the dust, or filibuster for fourteen hours on the state Senate floor.

Listening to that truth and responding to it isn't always easy, but it's free of that murky feeling in your heart that tells you to close the door, pull down the blinds, and bury yourself in pizza.

Respecting your body in this way means meeting physical and

emotional pain with purposeful remedies: movement, breath, suste-nance, friendship, and outreach. Discomfort is a signal. It's an open door. You can step through it or spend the rest of your life banging your head into a theoretical doorjamb. Staying stuck is a not-so-helpful option, and emotional eating and denial are prison cells wor-thy of a jailbreak.

• • •

My shoulder is doing much better, but not because of time or rest. The doctor thinks it's torn and will probably need surgery someday, but first I have to use it again. I have to continue to push through my own resistance and take the injured joint beyond where it wants to go. I made so many adaptations for the pain for so long that the mus-cles aren't functioning properly anymore. If he operated now, I would probably never get back to a normal range of motion.

Physical disobedience is about defying not only external forces but our own physical and emotional pain by meeting them with re-petitive acts of healing—even if that healing hurts like a son of a bitch.

For me, self-care can sometimes mean reaching for a top cabinet just like I would if my shoulder didn't hurt. Use it or lose it.

Over the past few months, I have stretched like it was a religion, praying to the shoulder gods and the pain gods and the gods of re-demption and healing five times a day. And then I have rested and iced and waited. Persistence and consistency are essential. Some days, I feel almost normal. Other days, the pain is back in force. The key, through it all, is maintaining an awareness of the tiny turning points—when I have it in me to push through and when I don't.

I can lift a jug of water with my right hand to stay safe, or do it with my left, carefully, mindfully, but effectively. Recognizing when to push and being willing to face the fire to get moving again are cru-cial. But sometimes I can't. I just can't lift the jug. It hurts too much, or I'm scared because my neck is also hurting that day. So on those days I don't, because it would do more harm than good. Most of the time, though, avoidance only makes the situation worse. It's a theme I've noticed throughout my life. I miss out when I fall into an avoidance mind-set: avoiding the sweat, avoiding the soreness, avoiding the awkwardness of a new class or an uncomfortable conversation. My muscles get stronger when they are challenged, of course, and weaker when they are neglected—and so does my mind.

We can't avoid pain, psychological or physical. We can choose to move through it or live with it. Those are the choices. We can't escape our bodies either. We can make use of what we've got, or waste our lives loathing these flesh and bone contraptions that make everything possible. Being alive, we get to experience taste, touch, and awareness. We can feel love, surprise, joy, and sadness. Are we really going to discount all of that because of a number on the scale? This is it. The only time we've got. The only bodies we've got.

Don't waste your time.

• • •

A friend of mine, Anna, is practicing how to take her physical space as well. She has been in a relationship for three years with a woman she loves. The two of them are happy and raising a daughter together. Anna has her own business with numerous employees, and she has lost fifty pounds in the last ten years. But, even with all of that going for her, she has a hard time appreciating her body and how much she has to offer. She can't see how smart, generous, and beautiful she is, but she does recognize that her self-image isn't what it should be.

She has been getting a series of massages as a kind of therapeutic exposure to unmask her body and flip the script in her mind. "I like to get massages from people I don't know well," she says. "It desensitizes me from feeling unattractive or untouchable. The more I let go of hiding myself from people, the more confident I feel that they don't hate or judge me for how my body looks. I find this infinitely easier to do with strangers than people I know. It's most difficult for me to be naked in front of my partner. It's terrifying that she might think my body is as ugly as I think it is."

Anna tells a heartbreaking story but a familiar one. Many women prefer the lights off in the bedroom to hide from their partners. Massage is a way for her to practice being anonymously okay with her body. It's a start. She can play with that feeling of abandon through the eyes and hands of a stranger. She can play with it when no one is around, too, and maybe someday she will turn on the light and let her partner love her as she is. On the surface, she is struggling with her body, but in reality, she's facing a much bigger question.

She is looking at a larger choice about whether to believe, in her own heart, that her external appearance defines her value. As long as she buys into that assumption, she will always be constrained, bound and gagged by a little bit of loose skin here or a touch of cellulite there.

Rejecting that premise is at the very heart of "liberty and justice for all." All of us. We all deserve respect as human beings. It is our birthright. We deserve it one hundred pounds overweight or thirty pounds underweight. We deserve it dark or light skinned. We deserve it disabled or able-bodied, and we deserve it male or female. We only squander that right by being thoughtless and unkind. It is not dependent on the nature of our bodies. We have to plant the flag of acceptance—firmly in the ground for ourselves—before we can demand that respect from those around us.

LET YOUR BODY BE

In 1999, US women's national soccer player Brandi Chastain hit a penalty kick that won the World Cup. She fell to her knees and tore off her jersey in a pure expression of ecstasy, revealing a sports bra beneath. My mother was horrified. I was up on my feet.

It's almost quaint now, but I don't think that moment caught fire like it did because of the bra exposure. It was the sheer, raw, athletic bliss burning its way out of a woman's body that was disconcerting and fascinating. Women's bodies don't take that kind of jurisdiction. They stay in place.

Consider taking physical jurisdiction in small or large portions of your day—five minutes today, ten tomorrow—being bold and unrepentant in your body.

Build it up like a muscle. Catch yourself shrinking, and align your posture instead. Study what it feels like to sink into your body, not only to own it, but to luxuriate in it.

It's always possible to get in better shape if that's what you want to do (and it can feel amazing), but if you don't want to do that, the only other viable option is to accept your body and love it *as it is* for all of the miraculous things it can currently do. The alternative is downright abusive. Love your body or do something to care for it, but don't go around hating it.

I choose not to play the part of a contortionist anymore.

When I dress for the airport, I will wear what makes me comfortable: warm enough, cool enough, easy walking shoes.

When I am sick as a dog and making the tenuous trip to the drugstore where I may or may not vomit all over the floor, I will not put on jeans and pull my hair back like a reasonable person because I am not in a reasonable state. I will go as I am in stinky sweatpants and get what I need. I would advise getting out of my way.

When I am dressing for a glamorous evening out (because, of course, that happens all the time), I will choose a dress or pants that flatter, that feel like beauty and strength on that day in that body. Shoes? Wedges. Fabulous, but comfortable.

When I am tired midafternoon, I will step away for however long I can to mainline fresh air and sunlight. I will plank when I'm pissed, and take off running when I need to break out. I will eat tater tots when I have been thinking about them for a week, and I will make fruit salad on Saturday mornings in the summer. And nobody can stop me.

I'd like to say I'll never again wear an item of clothing because I know the person I'm meeting will be dressed a certain way, that I will never again eat to sooth an aching heart, but those would be lies. I'm not all the way there yet, but I'm mighty close. I'm listening to my body and letting it be strong, tired, slim, puffy, achy, energized, or at peace. And that, in and of itself, is a glorious act of defiance.

• • •

How many times have you had the thought: *My business/love life would be better if I could get my body in shape?* Or the other way around: *My body would be in better shape if my business/love life was in order?* Which comes first? Does your body make you more capable of a successful life, or does a successful life make it easier to stay healthy? It's a catch-22, a chicken-and-egg scenario that can leave you paralyzed at one giant, multidirectional intersection. You run down one street for a few feet before turning on your heels to run down another, and then yet another. Work! Family! Romance! School! Friends! Volunteer! Student loans! Exercise! It's a schizophrenic existence, but at the center of the intersection is your body. It is present and accounted for no matter which road you're running down.

So when you find yourself at wit's end and you don't know which way to turn, the only thing to do is sit down on the curb with a bottle of water and a handful of almonds, to limber up and dust off for the next leg of the journey. If you keep running blindly in the same direction, you are running away from your center of gravity, and you will eventually break down, dehydrated, starving, and disoriented. But if you return to your body, back to home base, to refuel and check your location, you'll know exactly where you are and where to go next.

A REVOLUTION IN FEELING FINE

This planet is smack in the middle of a big, fat turning point of its own, and we need to be as durable and vocal as possible to help it settle into itself, nice and cozy. The expectations of our bodies that we've been living with for the last few centuries aren't going to fly for a society where women are leading the charge to save the planet and everyone on it. We are not programmed to recede or acquiesce. We know too much about what needs to be done. We face daunting situations every day, whether that means learning a new line of work or picking up a heavy water jug with an injured arm—but the small choices to feed our bodies with food, exercise, rest, and play prepare us for bigger turning points, which shape not only our individual lives but also the world we live in.

If you ask the women in your immediate circle about *their* turning points, you will hear stories about adaptation and ingenuity that will inspire you to return to your body—your center of gravity—and head out again, refreshed and ready.

You will hear stories of women like Meg Giuffrida, who has lived many lives at the age of forty-nine. She worked as a graphic designer and art director for twelve years. She has opened and closed three restaurants. She was the director of food services at a nonprofit community center, where she made 800 meals a day for children and seniors living in extreme poverty. She has been a Montessori teacher and an administrative assistant. She also started a culinary job-training program for people who couldn't find work because of felony convictions, and now she runs a bakery. She never completed college herself but says she loves to learn.

"I have blazed my own trail," she told me. "Where many people would have seen failure or been discouraged, I created opportunity. That's not to say I have never thought, 'Geez, what am I going to do now?' But I'm not afraid to take a risk, and I'm totally okay acknowledging when something is not working. I can always do what I need to do in the meantime to get by. I'm like a big, giant snowball collecting skills. I don't ever have the fear that I'm not going to have a next thing. I don't know what it will be, but it will be something. I'm comfortable with who I am, what I can do, and what I can give to people. I do things with gusto. I'm great on a camping trip or in a zombie apocalypse."

• • •

The zombie apocalypse is upon us. May we form armies of giant snow-balls, accumulating skills to bury the living dead, debilitating them and their savagery under mountains of beautiful, sparkling snow.

There isn't time anymore to wait for the powers-that-be to make decisions that are good for them—and for the rest of us. There's no time to waste worrying about triangles on our hips and rolls on our stomachs. There's no time for posing, and no time for food that makes us sick and foggy. The stakes are too high.

Our bodies serve our lives. They serve humanity, and they merit more than a cursory judgment by a stacked jury, holding them up like Christmas ornaments in comparison to each other. Our bodies de-serve the best we can offer at every turning point. And it starts with each of us—alone in a room or splayed out on the beach—in our bod-ies, feeling fine about every one of our parts, even the squishy ones.

◇◇

Fill in the Fact

Weird ways I contort my body to hide "flaws" are _____
_____.

When I notice myself doing this: _____, I'll
do this instead: _____.

An emotional or physical pain I feel regularly is _____
_____.

When I feel that pain, I will respond by _____
_____.

One insecurity I am ready to not give a damn about anymore is

_____.

The best thing about my body is _____

_____.

I hereby no longer give a rat's ass what _____

_____ thinks about my body.

◇◇◇

Catch yourself mannequin-twisting,
and sink into an even stance. We
can't be grounded in the world if
we aren't grounded in our bodies.

CHAPTER 13

Fragility as a Practice

When I was in college, I took a tai chi class from a professor named Felix Ivanov. He was in his fifties at the time, a product of the Russian theatre, physical comedy, clowning, stage combat, and character dance. He is a stout man, around five foot nine inches if I remember correctly. He had a big Santa Claus belly and a habit of humming classic rock songs in high-pitched tones under his breath with an occasional line popping out in English. *Everybo-dee must get stoned.* When my classmates and I arrived at class, we would not be surprised to find him wrestling with an imaginary foe like David slaying Goliath. Or he might be moving through a series of gentle tai chi movements, a process not complete until he was good and finished, no matter how many nineteen-year-olds were staring at him from the side of the room. He didn't like to wear shoes and was known to spend mornings in the park, swinging nunchucks around in a meditative dance that can only be described as adorable. He taught me never to drag a chair across the floor. *Pick it up. Put it where it goes. Be purposeful with all things, and never lock your knees. You must always be ready.*

For what, I wasn't sure.

One day in class, we were standing in a large athletic gym with high ceilings, waiting for Felix to give instructions. He was half-singing, half-talking in broken English about our next exercise, when a heavy steel beam fell from the ceiling directly on his head. His knees gave in like rubber, his body responding as if he knew it was coming. He dropped about six inches, allowing the beam to bounce off his head onto the floor and proclaimed, "Mmm, blumps!" He shook his head for a moment to get his brain back in place and continued on with a twinkle in his eye.

I will never forget the sight of that beam falling, and I will never again forget not to lock my knees.

· · ·

Strength is a primary focus of this book, but there is a huge difference between building strength and becoming hard.

When we are hard, we are much more vulnerable to dents.

We can't keep horrible things from happening, but we can be pliable and ready to move with whatever comes. In order to be durable under pressure, we will need to soften our knees. We can endure anger, uncertainty, and sadness without letting it break us *if* we can allow heartache to exist alongside resolve.

When barbaric laws are passed and enforced, when people in power are abusive or dismissive, we have a choice before us. We can rage and spit in the faces of politicians, for which they will label us irrational and out of control, or we can rebound like Simone Biles on a floor routine, meeting violence and hatred with openhearted determination.

In psychology, this kind of response is called noncomplimentary behavior. In the fight for civil rights, it is known as nonviolent resistance. When your neighbor goes ballistic for no reason, instead of escalating the conflict, you drop off a six-pack and tell her you'd like to find a way to solve what's bothering her. When the opposition at a rally turns aggressive and angry, you offer them bottles of water and handheld fans that double as bubble machines. It's hard for people to lash out when there is nothing to lash out against, and if they turn to violence, they are the ones that end up in jail or, at the very least, looking like numbskulls on Channel 4.

Gandhi, Martin Luther King Jr., Cesar Chavez, and Nelson Mandela all adopted this approach to oppression. In 1959, Martin Luther King Jr. and his wife, Coretta, traveled to India on what he referred to as a "pilgrimage" to learn from Gandhi's methods of nonviolent resistance. Before leaving the country at the end of the trip, he gave a speech on the radio saying, "since being in India, I am more convinced than ever before that the method of nonviolent resistance is the most potent weapon available to oppressed people in their struggle for justice and human dignity."[1]

When civil rights protesters were beaten with batons in the 1960s, pushed back with tear gas and water cannons, and in some cases shot and killed, an outcry arose nationwide, and between 1964 and 1968, the Civil Rights Act, the Voting Rights Act, and the Fair Housing Act were all signed into law. The people who suffered for that movement did not do so in vain. Their willingness to be vulnerable highlighted their humanity and revealed the brutality of the people attempting to silence them. They kept marching and sitting in. They continued raising their voices and won important protections—early victories—though many more battles were to come.

Long before Gandhi's tactics became famous, suffragettes in the United States and United Kingdom were employing methods of nonviolent resistance. At the first women's rights convention in the United States, at Seneca Falls in 1848, a resolution was passed in support of women's suffrage. It took *seventy-two* more years before American women got the right to vote in 1920. During that time, advocates for women's rights marched and organized. They were denigrated and arrested. They went on hunger strikes in prison and were force-fed. But they mobilized effective lobbying campaigns and moved their cause forward state by state. Only a few generations have passed since then. Clearly we have a long way to go. Women's history in this country reaches far beyond the singular issue of suffrage, but lessons of the past reverberate into the present. They are guideposts, hard evidence that determination to fight and willingness to be fragile are an explosive and effective combination.

When we fight with nonviolence, we claim the moral high ground while people promoting cruelty grow weaker by the day, exposed for their pettiness. Vulnerability can be the truest form of courage, the ultimate weapon to reveal callous, selfish behavior for what it is.

• • •

But fragility and nonviolence are not just tools for political progress. They are potent tools for personal progress as well. We do violence to ourselves by denying the needs of our bodies, and we devalue the benefits of being well when we ignore the brittle nature of our own health.

We, as living creatures, are inherently fragile. Our bodies are both delicate and finite. It's a hard truth but one that can make our lives more meaningful and vital. The layer between life and death is thinner than we would like to think, but as palliative care counselor Stephen Jenkinson says in the documentary *Griefwalker,* "Grief is the awakening. Grief is the sign of life stirring towards itself."

I learned from Mr. Jenkinson that in order to truly love something, you have to love the end of it as well—whether that means a career, a relationship, a life, or an illusion. Everything ends. The question is how we choose to process that fact. Do we go into denial and pretend it isn't happening? Or do we allow ourselves to stretch through and beyond our grief, permitting that grief to reignite signs of life?

We are living in the death of one era and into the life of another. This particular ending—of a time when too many of us (white women in particular) wrongfully believed that progress was on the march with or without our personal efforts—has left us bereft. It has stripped us of the illusion that we have dominion over our own bodies and that the most vulnerable among us—the elderly, refugees, children in poverty, and the disabled—will be protected by the basic functions of government.

We can't deny the suffering that comes with loss, but we can bend with the pain, arch our backs, and return to standing.

Trees grow stronger in response to the wind, and their roots grow deeper. This moment in history may feel like it's planted in the path of a category 5 hurricane. It has ripped us up, but it has also rooted us, weaving us together beneath the surface of the ground and leaving us stronger than ever. We can grieve the loss while, at the same time, falling madly in love with what it has mobilized within us: caring, grace, companionship, openness, and uncensored, outspoken truth telling. Dying can teach us a great deal about living.

LIVING WITH GRIEF

I spent three days last year at an immersion course in mindful care-giving at the Zen Hospice Project in San Francisco to explore death and what can be learned from it. The hospice grew out of the San Francisco Zen Center in 1987 as a response to the AIDS crisis, providing care for sick patients who could not find help elsewhere due to the heightened climate of fear. For nearly thirty years, the hospice staff has been running a beautiful, six-bed facility in a Victorian row house in a residential neighborhood in the center of San Francisco, providing twenty-four-hour nursing care for chronically ill and dying patients. They also train volunteers who offer daily, compassionate bedside care to a sixty-bed facility at Laguna Honda Hospital in the Bay Area. The course I attended is part of an ongoing community outreach to educate clinicians, family members, and the public about the comfort and healing that can be found in the shared human experience of dying.

The in-house chef bakes cookies or bread every day, whether the residents can eat them or not, because the smell is an experience everyone can cherish. Nurses on-site usher the patients and their families from living to dying to living again. They offer medical support to help the residents' bodies function optimally (bathing, feeding, and managing pain), but the staff takes no measures to prolong patients' lives. "There are no emergencies in hospice. There is nothing 'wrong' here," they told me.

The volunteers are trained to see and hear the patients, to treat them like regular people, rather than people who are halfway dead. Nobody wants to be reduced to a frightening reminder of the grim reaper knocking at the door. The patients want to be connected for as long as they can and to leave celebration and recognition behind in their wake.

I learned a lot that weekend in San Francisco. I faced up to the virtual reality pipe dream that I have control over when endings—either physical or existential—might come to me or to the people I love. Change is both blunt and inevitable, and death just happens to be the sharpest reminder of that fact. I was reminded to let death be death in the same way I let winter be winter. Not much of a choice there.

The message the hospice hopes to convey is not that people shouldn't get upset or experience fear or sadness in response to loss, but that we can flex with those experiences instead of lashing out against them or letting them consume us. If we allow life and everything in it to be in flux, we are allowing for growth, change, and sorrow to exist together, all at once. Beyond that, the greatest contribution we can make is to help our bodies and our loved ones' bodies do what they need to do in order to feel well.

With our physical bodies at ease, we are better able to serve, to function, and to show up when we are needed, fists raised in unison in nonviolent protest over a sea of living, breathing bodies—wide-awake and as loud as we damn well please.

• • •

When my father was diagnosed with pancreatic cancer at sixty-eight years old, we believed he had less than a year to live. Pancreatic is a particularly vicious kind of cancer with a survival rate of only 7 percent at five years. So far, he has made it two. I am not among the grieving yet, at least not in the way one does when a parent passes away, but grief has cast enough of a shadow to make my days softer than they were before, less addled with tiny triggers.

The week after his diagnosis, I returned home from visiting my parents out of state and needed to restock food in our kitchen. I got in my car and drove to the grocery store. At least I thought I was going to the grocery store, but when I pulled into a parking space and looked up, I realized that I had driven to the drugstore instead. I was lost. I shut off the engine and cried in that parking lot like he was already gone. I howled with the weight of the news for five, ten, fifteen minutes until the wave passed. Eventually, I turned on the car again and drove a whisper of myself to the grocery store, where I wandered around, examining the other shoppers and staff, wondering if they were grieving, too, wondering if they knew that death hovers so close.

I felt like a creature from the deep for months. When someone you love is dying, it can feel like you're walking around with a glass jar over your head, like the whole world is going on around you, oblivious to how fragile it all is, how prone to change with a single phone call, diagnosis, or wrong turn. But over time, Dad's treatments succeeded. Scans came back clear, and the shadow of impermanence moved further away. I found myself getting lost again in deadlines, meetings, and school events, but the edge of the shadow has remained with me—and I am so thankful for what it has brought. It has loosened my grip on the way things are "supposed to be" and allowed them to be as they are—messy, unpredictable, and poignant. It has made the truth matter more and other people's good opinions matter less. It has mellowed my days, making them lighter. And it has made the rage that dwells in my heart at the thought of the environment boiling and kids being denied healthy school lunches for political expedience a little bit more palatable. The shadow of death has created a place for me to hold anxiety—in a satchel at my side, attached to my body but apart from it.

● ● ●

We all have personal grief, and political grief, too. Both are natural and critical to living fully, but both can have a disastrous impact on our bodies if we don't know how to handle them.

I watch my clients going through tough times. At least one or two that come through my door every day are buried in stress or working to recover from trauma. Some sink into destructive behavior. They start to eat late at night, pound fast food, isolate themselves, or turn to substance abuse. But others let the grief wash over them like a rainstorm. They stand exposed to the storm. They accept circumstances for what they are and keep a steady eye on the many ways they can support the needs of their bodies, to continue growing stronger in the middle of the downpour. They carry on with fractured but gracious hearts and end up wiser and more peaceful than ever as the shadow moves back to the periphery of their lives.

The more we can release the illusion of control and accept the inevitability of the deluge, the better we will float, the more we will appreciate the lives and connections we still have, and the easier it gets to find a foothold at the center of the flood. Knocked off our feet and swept away, we can stretch our legs through the muddy water to reach solid ground beneath and find ourselves upright again as the clouds part and the earth begins to dry.

When the news is horrifying and we have understood the basic facts of a tragedy, we can turn off the twenty-four-hour coverage and take a walk and a deep breath and return home to wrap our arms around our kids, pets, lovers, or friends.

When we notice that a committee at work, school, or church is skewed toward a particular demographic, we can name it and find relief in ending the silence around race and economic class. We can reach out to our neighbors for help to diversify the institutions that support our communities.

We can speak truthfully. We can exercise and feed our bodies, and we can connect.

Then, whatever comes, we will still be standing here in living, breathing opposition to racism, sexism, bigotry, and greed. We will be here until we're not, and that's okay, too. But while we still have these bodies at our disposal, can we please make use of them? And enjoy them? And treat them as if they matter?

ENDURANCE

One of my clients is a forty-two-year-old manager of a retail store. Her husband loads boxes at a big box warehouse. They have an eight-year-old daughter and a diabetic dog. Her husband is a high-functioning alcoholic who has confessed to a long-term affair with a high school sweetheart. He claims the affair is over and that the drinking is under control, but there are empty bottles hidden throughout the house and no one really knows the status of the tryst. He has liver problems and sleep apnea but refuses to see a doctor for lack of money and lack of will. My client runs the household, pays for everything, makes sure their daughter gets what she needs for school, works full-time, and manages the stress of never knowing which husband she will get on any given day—the one who is outside playing jump rope or the one who is passed out cold on the sofa. But she loves him. They have been together for twenty years. He is the father of her daughter and the love of her life. There isn't a day that goes by that she doesn't think of leaving him, but she stays. Those reasons are hers. The trade-off is something only she can understand. What might lie on the other side of a decision to end their marriage is unknown. It could be liberating or just as difficult and far lonelier.

But the wear and tear on her body is obvious when things get bad. The relationship is not what she imagined it would be when they got married, and the life they have is not what she wanted. She mourns that loss. It hangs over her like a slow-growing cancer. Maybe she will beat it. Maybe she won't. Either way, her body is the only permanent home she's got, and, thankfully, she has chosen to make her body a priority, a place of respite.

In the past two years, she has quit ginger ale in exchange for water and tea. She takes walks outside for ten minutes every day on her lunch break. She has filled her desk with grapes, oranges, and nuts to steer clear of a nasty chip addiction, and when she is at the end of her patience, with anxiety spiking and nowhere to turn, she drops for a set of push-ups. Grounded, she gets up again and keeps going. "Self-care is the only reliable stability I have," she says. "I don't know what I would do if I didn't have those tools in place. I would be a total mess right now if I were still turning to Doritos for comfort. I know how to take care of myself now, so I can deal with all of this other crap."

We can't always be strong, but we can be persistent and adaptable. We can put one foot in front of the other, doing whatever it takes to keep our bodies functioning and our vision clear. Without that, we can't accomplish much of anything.

History shows that perseverance and nonviolent resistance work, but we have to keep showing up. And we can't show up if we are broken in half by depression or the physical repercussions of stress.

We are fragile and angry. We are horrified by current events that strike at the heart of our belief in common decency. We are bereaved, but that anger and sorrow flows from deep, abiding love for our fellow human beings. We are grieving because we care, and our hearts are more awake than ever.

The death of indifference is a good thing. We can find a lot to love there.

Over the last fifty years, while minority communities around the country were working for recognition and an equal shot, some of the rest of us were coasting along, riding the wave of the blood, sweat, and tears invested by the civil rights and feminist activists of the 1960s and 1970s and those who proceeded them. We shrugged off the pay gap and our astonishing underrepresentation in government, assuming these problems would correct themselves over time, but they have not.

We get it now. We have been slapped in the face and moved to take a stand. Many of us are ready to do our part, following on the heels of those who have been at it all along. We are ready to speak out publicly and soften our stance as bullies start throwing punches, knowing full well that we are not alone and reinforcements will be coming from all sides.

Love can transcend this death of indifference if we allow the death to be an inherent part of a new beginning. The bounce that follows a crushing blow can lift us to even greater heights.

We are at our most powerful right now because we are no longer blind, no longer hanging on to false truths.

We are united in the conviction that the current state of affairs cannot stand. Our job going forward is to mend the holes in the safety net that hangs in tatters beneath us. Let the deluge come. Let it all come. We will be right here, arm in arm through birth and death and everything in between.

Something has died, and it stinks to high heaven. We need to bury it and issue last rites, so we can get on with the work of birthing something new.

We're going to need our strength, every last bit of it, kept afloat by the residue of loved ones lost and well-meant idealism shattered. Eat your vegetables. Keep moving, and don't forget not to lock your knees.

$$\diamond$$

Fill in the Fact

A situation where I feel triggered or antagonized is _____

_____.

I can meet it with nonviolent resistance by _____

_____.

When I am grieving a loss or defeat, I will persist by _____

_____.

An ending or death I am ready to accept is _____

_____.

A physical place I can visit to heal and recharge is _____

_____.

◇◇

We can't deny the suffering that
comes with loss, but we can
bend with the pain, arch our
backs, and return to standing.

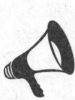

CHAPTER 14

Keep It Interesting

When I was a little girl, I read the story of Peter Pan. I read about Wendy's flights of fancy and her punishment of being removed from the nursery because it was time for her to grow up. I read about Peter's solution to take her to Neverland where she could be a mother to the Lost Boys and tell them stories. And in the end, I read about her resentment at being reduced to cooking and carrying wood with the squaws rather than dancing and chanting with the boys.

I heard that story in many different forms, but it never occurred to me to resent Wendy's treatment. It didn't seem anything other than normal. It was just another in a long line of stories with male protagonists taking on the world while the girls were relegated to secondary story lines.

I didn't get angry. In fact, I didn't consciously associate myself with Wendy at all. I had no interest in sewing or mothering and set about to prove it. In my mind, I wasn't Wendy. I was Peter, reckless and forever young, unconcerned with rules and other such antiquities. I was determined not to be any of the things a girl was supposed to be. Throughout high school and college, I made it my business to be one of the boys—a pursuit that unintentionally put all of my focus on impressing them, entertaining them, and consistently holding their opinions above my own.

The most direct route to their good graces was, of course, through my body, offering it up as a plaything or a tease. The race was on to lure them in by being small and delicate and to throw them off by being wild and unaccountable. Meanwhile, I ignored or alienated my female peers and completely disregarded any wisdom my mother had to share.

I wanted to be chosen. By the men. I wanted to be seen, but only in the right light. I didn't realize yet that I could be a woman and a whole person at the same time and that the companionship and insight of the women around me would become one of the most cherished gifts I could ever hope for.

I grew up in the 1980s and 1990s, not exactly olden times, but my family was strict. I was forbidden to call boys on the telephone because they were supposed to initiate every conversation, and there was certainly not to be any sex before marriage. Both of those well-laid plans fell flat. I had no intention of meeting those expectations and experienced them like a straightjacket, accessorized with a generous roll of duct tape wrapped around my nose and mouth. I felt suffocated, but the illicit phone calls I made to little boys as a ten-year-old girl, the unsatisfying sex I had as a teenager, and the randy photos I took for my Americana band when I was in my twenties did not break me out of the prison of feminine expectvations that I was trying to escape. They locked me in deeper. The steel bars of my cage were all built around sex and my female body, so I took those on as the front lines of battle.

Unfortunately, by trying to break my body free, I objectified it even more, playing the vamp instead of the mother. The first fifteen years of my young adult life were built in reaction to those expectations, which left me with very little regard for my own truth and what I had to offer. Who did I want to be? What kind of person? Confident? Intelligent? Did I want to be an attorney? A veterinarian? A photographer? A reporter? An engineer? An architect? A designer?

No, no. I wanted to be a statue, with a dancer's body. I wanted to never, ever have gas. I wanted to be three sizes smaller and two inches shorter than I was and aspired to never be caught eating in public. Smoothies were okay, but chewing was unseemly.

Give me booze and sex and a copy of *Crime and Punishment,* and I'll raise you one. Give me a sandwich, and I'll have to excuse myself for a panic attack.

It wasn't until I felt like a thoroughly used up piece of trash that I decided to stop abusing my body by fasting in public and binging in private, deriding the image I saw staring back at me in the mirror, and hoping that my many disguises were working.

Instead, I hiked up a hill. And hiked again and again until I could breathe again. And once I could breathe again, I could see and think again. And when I could think again, I thought, *That guy's an asswipe. What the hell am I doing?* And I was alone again, and I thought, *This job is mind-numbing.* And I went back to school, and started a business, and wrote for no reason, and met a guy who saw me as a whole person, and built a life in a part of the country I never expected and in a traditional way I never imagined.

ENTERTAINMENT AND ADVOCACY: A WELCOME DISTRACTION

The stories we are told as children shape us. Whether we work to emulate them or act out against them, they mold who we become as adults. I grew up believing that women's liberation was a thing that had already been done. It happened when women got the vote and when hippies burned their bras, long before I was born. The story in history class was that women were equal and the fight was over, but the story I saw all around me was that women were either chaste and devoted or they were Cherry Pie, ripe and sticky.

I wanted to be Peter Pan, but as a woman the only expression of that lively abandon that I could see was to flaunt my sexuality in ways that had nothing to do with my own desires and everything to do with the desires of the men around me. I was aggressively, unwittingly re-acting to Wendy's plight, and I sacrificed my body in the process.

I don't have a daughter, but I do have a son growing up in this new era of intentional girl power. Nashville had a female mayor for the first few years of his life and, between her and the mayor on *Paw Patrol*, I discovered that my son thought mayors were *always* women and never men. He watches *Doc McStuffins*, about an African American girl who plays doctor to broken toys in her playhouse clinic. He adores *Word Girl* and sees strong female leads in films like *Moana* and *Zootopia*. He isn't old enough to see *Wonder Woman* 2017, but I'm waiting for the day that he is.

Unfortunately, portrayals of men and boys in movies and cartoons are not advancing as rapidly as those for girls, with images of violence and disinterest still isolating young men from their essential human vulnerability. It's a blind spot in popular culture that's a disservice to our guys and the women they love and respect.

My family remedies this, at least in part, with a visit to the Pride Parade every year, where my son waves a flag, proudly sporting his sequined rainbow fedora. The parade exposes him to many of the strongest men I know, both gay and straight, who loudly support values of kindness, acceptance, and unity. He will become more aware of discrimination and bias as he gets older, of course, but times have changed. Gender identity is magnificently fluid in a way it has never been before.

As I look around at little kids marching in step with their parents to defend human rights and coloring postcards to send to their senators about school funding, I am filled with faith in the future. As I watch young women not only accepting their bodies, but championing them, I am overcome with relief. These kids are surrounded with an onslaught of positive images and role models that my peers and I never dreamed of seeing.

Sometimes these new portrayals of women can seem heavy-handed, especially when produced by corporations trying to capitalize on this age of enlightenment. And, of course, there are still stereotypes being perpetuated around the world and all over the internet of women as pawns for men's pleasure, but those stereotypes look increasingly archaic. They would be funny if they weren't so insidious. Positive changes in the common wisdom are in their infancy, not yet fully formed. We need women in positions of power throughout the entertainment industry so the decisions about those portrayals can come from authentic, informed, female perspectives. The changes are slow and awkward, but we are unquestionably blessed to be living in the midst of a magnificent tidal wave of pro-woman, pro-minority pop culture.

Influential women like Samantha Bee, America Ferrera, Beyoncé, Shonda Rhimes, Geena Davis, Lena Waithe, Reese Witherspoon, Amy Poehler, Jenji Kohan, and Lena Dunham are making thoughtful works of art that empower women by portraying them as candid, spirited, and complicated.

Thanks to these women and many more, by the time our kids grow into themselves, their expectations for their positions in society will be fundamentally different than ours were and dramatically different than those of their grandparents. The ways we bring them up at home will have a lot to do with what expectations they hold, but change also inevitably seeps in from the stories they hear and the content they consume. Hopefully, these girls won't ever have to close their eyes, turn their heads, and pretend to be somewhere they're not. They will know that they can push away and establish themselves on their own terms.

A whole new generation of activists is on the move. They have been mobilized, but it's up to us to keep them engaged and to keep *ourselves* engaged as well.

We live in a world of short attention spans. The majority of us are not ignorant or uninterested. We're exhausted and overwhelmed. Sometimes we just can't stand to hear any more debates. Kids and adults alike are thirsty for distraction, and the entertainment industry can play a crucial role in filling that need in strategic, thoughtful ways.

Musicians, artists, filmmakers, playwrights, novelists, television producers, journalists, and advertising art directors have the power to quench the thirst of young and older generations with ground-breaking portrayals of women and minorities as intelligent, intuitive, and decidedly equal members of society. Women don't always have to be superheroes on screen, and we certainly don't need to portray men as blockheaded simpletons. We need entertaining, challenging stories and music. We need something exciting to inform us, and something entertaining to keep us coming back for more.

It's up to us to create and support content that will change the way we think about ourselves and the world—and to have a good time doing it.

We can draw on the creative performers and artists we see making activist art and translate that into our own acts of resistance. We can learn from folks who go around glitter-bombing politicians in the name of LGBTQ rights and from the women dressed as "handmaids," protesting threats to reproductive rights at state and national capitol buildings.

Our responses to injustice don't always have to be deadly serious. What we're fighting for is serious, but our methods don't have to be. We will get far more attention and stick with the movement longer if we play around with our activism while musicians and writers are playing around with fresh inspiration for who we intend to be as a country and as individuals.

Entertainment is one of the most powerful weapons at our disposal. If we hope to persevere and win this fight, we need to loosen our grip a bit and have some fun with it. We need breast-pumping parties on the steps of every federal building in the country until they fully fund Medicaid. We need to offer up sippy cups of whole milk to our representatives on their way into and out of their offices every day until they stop acting like selfish, petulant children and agree to provide for the basic needs of the most vulnerable populations in our society. We need dance parties in congressional hallways, celebratory fund-raisers for progressive candidates, and doggy fashion shows outside polling places on Election Day. And we need to bring the kids along for all of it so they can see how we roll. It's time to fight fire with cheese whiz.

Of course, we need the truth. We need the unvarnished, disturbing truth about all the disasters unfolding before us. Statisticians, investigative reporters, and policy wonks should absolutely keep up the work of documenting the devastating impact of rollbacks in social support systems, deregulation of financial markets, proliferation of guns, sky-high incarceration rates, and a widening gap between rich and poor— but that lift is too heavy for most of us to bear every day. We have jobs and love affairs and kids with book reports. Most of us adults can barely keep up with the relentless flow of issues desperately in need of attention, and an avalanche of depressing data with no fun in sight is far more likely to dishearten young, energetic voters than it is to motivate them. We need the truth, and that truth is far from pretty. But once the truth is exposed, we have to find ways to amuse ourselves while getting the word out. This is going to be a long haul in the middle of a pitch-black night. We're gonna need glow sticks for the ride.

Fill in the Fact

An artist, filmmaker, or musician I love who is doing important work is _____.

I can help spread the word about her or him by _____

_____.

A cause I'm working for that could use a dose of entertainment is _____.

A playful way to fund-raise or connect that cause with new supporters is _____.

Portrayals I will no longer accept in my media diet are _____
_____.

◇◇

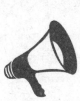

A whole new generation of
activists is on the move. They
have been mobilized, but it's up
to us to keep them engaged and
to keep *ourselves* engaged as well.

CHAPTER 15

Carry On

My mom and I grew up in very different times, and it's my understanding that, in hindsight, she realized that many of the limitations she put on me were holdovers from her own upbringing. We don't see eye to eye on a lot of things, but she did teach me, throughout my life, the far-reaching value of community. She taught me not to look away from other people's pain, to be present and make myself useful. She taught me that I am stronger when I'm standing arm in arm with people of every age, race, religion, gender, and income level and showed me, by example, that discouragement isn't the end of the line. She has been horrified by political injustice for many more years than I have been alive, but she never stopped reaching out to feed hungry people, to support young moms with a cup of tea and open ears, or to drive elderly immigrants to the doctor when they need someone to help translate frightening and unfamiliar medical language.

One of the greatest things she taught me was that the oldest people in the room are often the most interesting, that their wrinkled faces and stilted speech mask priceless insights. So when I thought about disobedience, about women holding fast and liberating themselves and their children one gutsy step at a time; when I thought about who sets examples and breaks barriers, I thought about the old ladies living quietly in houses and apartments throughout our neighborhoods. I wanted to know what they had to say about how life used to be and how far we've come.

• • •

I got on a plane on a cold February morning to try to find out. I went to see Lois Lee Frauchiger, a ninety-six-year-old woman who lives by herself in a small, brick ranch house, on a winding, tropical, tree-lined, dead-end street, on the outskirts of a small town in central Florida.

Lois was born in Cumberland, Maryland. Her dad worked at a tire factory, and her mom was a homemaker until, when Lois was a teenager, her mother fell into a railroad track and was killed by an oncoming train. After this early loss, Lois and her brother "Lefty" joined the effort in World War II. Lefty was deployed to exercise his skills with carrier pigeons while, at age twenty-two, Lois graduated in the first class of the Women's Army Corps in 1943. She served in the quartermaster service for three years, including a stint in New Guinea where a local tribal chief tried to buy her for the price of several pigs, a compliment of the highest accord. While there, she lived in a tent on base, commuting back and forth to her post where she redacted letters going back to the home front to prevent sensitive information from making it out to the public. To spruce up her tent, she built furniture out of discarded shipping boxes and says she "liked it just fine."

For her service, Lois was awarded a Philippine Liberation Ribbon, an American Campaign Medal, and a Women's Army Auxiliary Corp Ribbon. She rose to the rank of first lieutenant before coming back to the states, enrolling briefly at the University of Oklahoma, and marrying a widower whose wife had died in childbirth. He was left with a four-year-old son and a newborn baby girl, and Lois adopted them as her own. A few years later, she and her new husband, Fritz, completed the family with another baby girl.

Fritz worked for the US State Department as a linguist, where he was charged with developing language programs in France, Germany, Lebanon, Syria, Jordan, and Turkey during the 1950s and 1960s. Throughout this time, Lois was frequently left alone with the three children to navigate housing, schools, clothing, and food in countries where she could not speak the language and in some cases was not allowed to move freely. She never finished her studies or pursued a career of her own.

Her daughter told me that, overseas, Lois "developed a life philosophy of calmly accepting whatever is at hand, toughing it out, and never quitting." She was a dutiful State Department wife, rising above and beyond the tasks that were expected of Department employees' spouses during this era "to entertain, attend mandatory teas and other functions, and comport themselves to the satisfaction of the State Department." By 1970, Lois and Fritz returned to the United States and eventually relocated to Florida, where she assumed yet another set of roles as a university professor's wife, part-time librarian at the high school, and competitive amateur tennis player. She also took on the task of renovating the little ranch house where she lives today, an accomplishment in which she takes a great deal of pride.

I went to see Lois in hopes of finding some life-altering secret to her longevity and perseverance. I hoped she would point a clear spotlight on how to live long and well, how to handle the expectations placed on women while hacking away at the tangled, thorny brambles in our paths. But Lois wasn't interested in the brambles. She was more interested in the view.

I didn't find any epiphanies there. What I found was mundane in the best possible way.

I sat her down over a stack of scrapbooks and dredged up every painful detail from her past. I started by asking how she handled becoming a mom to two kids, basically overnight, at age twenty-five. "I just did it," she said. "It was my job, and they were great kids. I loved being a mom."

I asked how she survived two bouts of cancer: breast cancer in her fifties and lymphoma in her seventies. "My friends drove me to all of my chemo appointments," she replied. "We had a great time! It was great fun in the car."

"Did you fear for your life?" I asked.

"Oh, I don't know. I just figure what happens happens," she said. "There's not much you can do about that."

I pressed on, asking about the sudden death of her husband after fifty-one years of marriage and, the most devastating heartbreak of her life, the loss of her grandson at age thirty-three to a MRSA infection he likely acquired during a prison stay for heroin abuse.

She paused, looked over my shoulder, and said without a shred of bitterness, "I don't think much about any of that. I just like to sit and admire the lake."

I turned to look behind me—away from the folding card table where we sat and the dusty photo albums we had pulled out of the silent corners of her home—and saw for the first time what she had been looking at all morning. The rear wall of her unassuming, one-story house was a solid sheet of windows and sliding glass doors. Beyond the windows lay a small but beautiful lake with an enormous storklike bird, a great blue heron, standing nearly five feet tall, like a yard ornament, just a few feet from where we sat. Its massive wingspan stretched out over the water, and we watched it fly away.

That lake is her lifeblood. It gets her up every morning and feeds her all day.

I wanted Lois to lead me to the Fountain of Youth, to offer some great insight about the past and future. I asked if she had any message for people hoping to live long, happy, healthy lives.

She stood up slowly with her walker and shuffled into the kitchen. She opened a cabinet, pulled out a mug, and showed it to me. "Keep Calm and Carry On," it said.

Lois didn't want to think about the difficult parts of her life and how she got through them. All she really wanted to do was show me the lake.

She was trying to tell me to relax, that there are no secrets, that I could choose to live or squander a lifetime ruminating over things I couldn't control.

Lois raised two daughters and a son. She urged all the kids to pursue education and travel and encouraged them in their professional choices. She had the life she wanted. She didn't feel anything was left undone and didn't strain against the notion that she should center every choice around being a wife and a mom. She is at peace with the course of her life and secure in the legacy of strength and free-spiritedness she has passed down. She urged her daughters, in particular, to become financially independent. Both are now retired. One was a lawyer and the other taught English at Hong Kong University.

Lois's eldest great-granddaughter—let's call her Sage—is thirteen years old. Sage plays bass in two bands, mostly covers of funk, disco, and Latin music, but they plan to start writing original pop-punk songs soon.

I asked Sage what she thinks of when I say the word *beauty*.

She said, "I think of someone who is kind and caring, someone who knows how to take care of those around them while also being able to take care of and recognize their own feelings. I don't know if I'm beautiful like that. I hope so. I do what I can."

I asked how she feels about her body.

"I feel pretty okay in my skin," she said. "In my school, we're accepting about our bodies. We don't give a crap if you're fat or skinny or gay or whatever. You've just gotta be you. That's what matters. Being okay with yourself makes it a lot easier to be okay with others."

Sage would like to be a musician, actor, or writer someday, but she said, "If that doesn't happen, I'd like to be a forensic pathologist, and maybe live in London. I don't know. I'll let life unfold as it wants."

Patience and surrender so young.

Whether as a musician or a pathologist, this teenager is starting her life with an advantage many of us from earlier generations did not have. She is standing on two strong legs that she does not despise. She feels "pretty okay" in her body. I can barely imagine what it would have meant to be "pretty okay" in my body at the age of thirteen—or twenty-eight. I can barely imagine what I might have been able to accomplish. Sage and her generation are showing us exactly what is possible, how much can be accomplished when your values and passion matter infinitely more than pant size.

Lois's *come what may, do what needs to be done* attitude has made its way down through three generations of women, expanding exponentially. She spent a lifetime happily dedicated to being a caretaker, but at the heart of that dedication was a commitment to instill courage and independence in her children, all three of them.

We have Lois—and women like her—to thank for planting the seeds in our mothers' and grandmothers' minds that they didn't have to be "just" women. They could be people too.

· · ·

Down another country road, in North Carolina this time, I found seventy-five-year-old Linda Carl, a semiretired art expert with an insatiable appetite for travel. She has multiple sclerosis and has endured several crippling car accidents in recent years, but in spite of that, it's surprisingly difficult to track her down.

The first time I tried to reach her, she was piranha fishing in the Amazon rain forest in Peru. The second time, she was headed for a month in Mongolia. When I did nail down some time with her, I asked how she's taken care of her body over the years to maintain such a high activity level. "I have ice cream every night after dinner," she said. "*When in doubt, eat* is my motto. Food is important. Years ago when everyone else stopped eating butter, I never did. I never ate margarine. Nope. Never did. These days, when I'm tense, like with this last election, I get on the elliptical trainer and go faster than I normally go. I try to work it out. And when I can't sleep, I have a quarter of a cup of bourbon and read. It slows me down."

She said that the only time she ever gained weight and couldn't get it off was when she was dieting. "Now it looks so silly to me. I would skip lunch or have a very light lunch and then come back home and snack enormously."

She also told me that she likes to lead with the fact that she's Jewish. She doesn't practice but likes to "identify culturally so that anyone who doesn't want to like me because of it can go ahead and do that."

Twenty years younger than Lois, Linda had the benefit of her mother's example of public advocacy. Her mom worked at her dad's electrical supply company for many years before spearheading the Phoenix, Arizona, Council for Civic Unity, which desegregated the Phoenix school system in 1953, a year before the Supreme Court ruled on *Brown vs. Board of Education*. She also partnered with a local seamstress to start a back-to-school clothing drive, which still outfits thousands of children in Phoenix every year with backpacks, clothes, and shoes.

Building on her mom's example, Linda graduated from the University of California Berkeley in 1962, "before it got wild," and went against the times by continuing on with a master's degree from Berkeley and a PhD in adult and continuing education from the University of Illinois.

Like Lois, Linda married, had children, and taught them the unquestionable importance of intellectual and financial independence. She believes that if she had been just a few years younger, she could have benefited more from women's liberation. She is acutely aware that she has earned less than her male counterparts throughout her career. The discrepancy in her earning potential was obvious to her from a young age. As a kid, she remembers being frustrated that her brother was allowed to have a paper route while she was not. "It was something girls couldn't do. I didn't like it, but I accepted it. It was just the way things were."

The odds may have been against her all along, but Linda never bought into the roles she was expected to occupy or the limitations she was expected to adopt. She has spent the bulk of her career organizing immersive art courses and leading tours all over the world for adult students to study art, food, and culture throughout Asia and South America. The multiple sclerosis has robbed her of her balance and her favorite activity, bike riding, but if you ask her, it's no big deal.

"I haven't had any real problems," she said. "When I look back at how I handled hard times, I didn't dwell. My whole attitude toward life is that when a problem occurs, and it's right in front of you, deal with it. My modus operandi is to think about how I can deal with a situation, and then do it. I don't dwell on the future."

• • •

That kind of adaptable, *deal with it and move on* mind-set has served both Lois and Linda well, but I had to wonder if that approach was a luxury of privilege, at least to some degree. Both women are white. Neither has had an idyllic life. They have both moved through enormous challenges, and, as Linda mentioned, she has faced discrimination because of her Jewish heritage. But I wondered if that same philosophy of steady but flexible determination could hold true and serve people who have faced entrenched bias, based not only on gender but on skin color. I wondered, specifically, about the African American women who came up just a few years behind Linda at the axis of the civil rights movement, the first generation that integrated white schools in the South.

I found my answer in Joy Smith, who was the first black child to attend a school called Emma Clemons Elementary in Nashville, Tennessee, in 1957 at the age of six. She is now sixty-six years old and a theater director, storyteller, and actor in New York City.

Joy was kind enough to tell me her story, and it was one I needed to hear.

Her father was a well-known pastor at the forefront of the campaign for civil rights and president of the local chapter of the NAACP, and her mom was a teacher at Tennessee State University. They "joined twelve other black parents in filing suit in US District Court against the Nashville Board of Education" to force integration in the local school system, and, when the time came, they sent their little girl to the all-white school just a block from their home on her first day of first grade.[1]

The kids sang taunting songs. For years, Joy was disinvited from playdates, birthday parties, and the school's Brownie troop. Some of the boys sicked a dog on her once, and that first year in school, at six years old, she was called "nigger" for the first time when a friend's father discovered her standing in the stairwell of his home, looking for a kitten her friend had promised. Joy never got to see the cat. She was told "they threw the kittens out the window."

"That kind of thing happened all the way up through high school," she told me. "People said and did awful things. When I tell people about it now, they don't understand why I'm not angry, but it was just part of my life. The whole message of civil disobedience was about being nonviolent. I asked my mother once, 'Why don't the protestors fight back?' And she said, 'Because it puts you in the same category as the people who are doing terrible things to you.' And I've never forgotten that. I decided I had to find a way to deal with it because I'm not someone who fights. I didn't even think of fighting. So I decided to laugh at them. I figured it would make them feel ridiculous. And it worked. They usually stopped, which is all I wanted them to do."

When Joy was a senior in high school, she wrote a speech called *Soul* for a public-speaking competition. She started with the concept of soul within the African American community and expanded it to a greater human imperative "to be kind and understanding of different kinds of people. Soul isn't exclusive to any one culture," she said as she described that speech to me. "People are people. We're all in this together. You can't separate human rights issues. We all really want the same things. It's all about respect and tolerance and fairness. We should listen to each other, even if we disagree." She won the competition and landed at Wellesley College in 1970, the year after Hillary Clinton graduated.

Joy has continued to use laughter and the arts throughout her career to shed light on civil rights, class prejudice, and economic disparity wherever it can be found. For thirty years, she directed *Freedom Train*, a play for young audiences about Harriet Tubman and the Underground Railroad that has toured thousands of schools nationwide. And for even longer, she has been teaching music and storytelling from nursery schools to high schools, universities to retirement homes. She said, "Music and stories bring people together and help them feel better. They help people work through the issues that some of them face."

They have helped her through difficult times as well. Beyond the challenges of being a black woman in America, Joy has seen her fair share of heartache, in particular when she lost her husband to illness and became a widow in her thirties. Music has been her greatest solace. She plays guitar, piano, and sings—alone and in front of large audiences. It keeps her grounded, especially when she is ready to "fly off the handle." She works her body to handle stress, too. She started practicing yoga long before it was popular, and still practices daily.

Joy has lived through tumultuous times, but through all of them, she sang, told stories, and kept moving. As a white woman, I can only partly understand the discrimination that she and millions of minorities face in this country. When I worked as a cocktail waitress, I learned too well how it felt to be grabbed by handsy patrons who had a few too many drinks, but I never had anyone refuse to take a drink from me because of the color of my skin, or an employer refuse to hire me for that matter. So it is vital for me to hear stories like Joy's, to listen and try to understand and to consider the experiences we do and do not have in common.

I can't fully comprehend what she has been through, but according to Joy, we all have a lot more in common than we might think. She has been able to literally laugh in the face of adversity, to "deal with it and move on" in much the same way as Lois and Linda. I take tremendous inspiration from all of them. If they can keep calm and carry on after all they've seen, I can certainly do the same.

• • •

I got basically the same advice from all of the brilliant, older ladies I spoke with. I saw glimmers of bemusement and touches of pity in their eyes as I peppered them with unanswerable questions. The message they wanted to impart was simple.

Don't sweat the small stuff. It isn't worth a single minute of your time. Every moment, conversation, and political act doesn't have to be transcendent. Sometimes living, loving, and speaking the truth is the best you can do.

They stopped, a long time ago, worrying about how far they have come and how much further they have to go. Whether smashing boundaries or working within systems of marriage, motherhood, or industry, these women did not get bogged down in day-to-day drama or resentment. They had good old-fashioned moxie. They determined what could be done with the challenges they faced, and took whatever action they could. There was sadness and frustration along the way, but that's not where they chose to linger.

So those of us coming up now—who are not yet unstable on our bikes or pushing around walkers, who have not yet lost spouses or grandchildren—cannot fall to pieces in reaction to the news or even in reaction to our own personal challenges.

There is a place for shock. There is a place for grief. And there is always and forever a place for heartache, but when we turn all of that in on ourselves, we inflict more damage than the outside world ever could. We set ourselves back, and there is no place for that.

Of course, we get caught up in the enormity of the fight sometimes. It's too big for any of us to take on alone, and it's no surprise that we lose perspective on the purpose of taking care of our bodies. Why bother to keep our energy up? Why keep fighting to heal suffering in the world when the suffering seems so endless? Our individual efforts can feel like toilet paper in a tornado. Useless. And taking care of our own health and well-being can seem laughably unimportant in the midst of poverty, global warming, sex slavery, and so on.

Fixing something as minor as a frozen shoulder can seem like an almost worthless pursuit. But it's not. I'm 95 percent back to normal now. I can hold up my sign and lift my water jug almost pain-free, and that means I can take care of a lot of other important things that need attention.

Our bodies are everything. They are the tools that our mothers and their mothers used to end wars. Women have used their bodies to demand the right to vote, the right to work, the right to birth control, the right to safe working conditions, the right to choose, the right to equal funding for sports and education, the right to say "no," and the right to serve in any position in the armed services for which they are qualified.

Our bodies are agents of change.

Women have come a very long way in a very short period of time. We advanced so far, in fact, that many of us were lulled into believing that momentum would be enough to carry us forward. We got distracted while scraping by on maternity leave and negotiating extended payment plans on medical bills. A lot of us managed to get good jobs and solid educations, but many of us also fell through the cracks. And, overall, our accumulated wealth and influence suffered.

Our health has suffered as well. We are resilient creatures, but if we are subdued by heart disease, diabetes, obesity, anxiety, addiction, and depression, we will not have the physical strength to keep walking, tumbling, and protesting our way forward. If we are sick and tired, we will have no choice but to submit to public policies made by those already in power. Decisions about our bodies and lives and our children's lives will not be ours to make.

And no. That's not going to work.

We need to be on the board, on the panel, on the ballot, and behind the camera. Everywhere. With 51 percent representation.

This isn't a new objective. It's an old one in which we have made a lot of progress, but in the heat of battle, we've neglected one very important resource. The front lines are not in Washington, DC. They are at home—in our refrigerators and on the floors of our closets where our sneakers sit, ready for action. We're emerging from a tsunami of systemic injustice and shocking disregard for women's bodies and intellect. Don't take it into your heart.

The ways we view our bodies; the ways we move and feed them; the ways we dress and care for them are entirely up to us. Our thoughts and personal behavioral choices belong to us. This is one domain where we have all the power—should we choose to exercise it. Wellness allows us to live our lives fully, in bodies that feel accessible, balanced, and free of self-consciousness. It lets us get the job done without having to think twice about whether we're physically up to the challenge.

It's time to step off the tilt-a-whirl of despair, guilt, and self-destruction, get our footing, and make a run for it—up a hill in flat-footed Converse or naked feet—until we can learn to love our whole, entire bodies, until we can see the sky again.

• • •

At the end of my interview with Lois, I took her out to the edge of the lake in her wheelchair. She thought it might have been six months since she had been out there, just a hundred feet from her sliding glass door. When she was seated comfortably on a wooden bench by the water, I asked, "Can I take your picture? I collect pictures of people and things I think are beautiful." She blushed and straightened up in her geometric rainbow blouse. The wind blew her short, snow white hair back, and she grinned for the camera. Radiant.

The challenges ahead might seem overwhelming, but there is one fight we can win right now. We can join forces with our bodies. We can take them back for our own enjoyment and our own purposes.

We can listen to them and give them what they need, recognizing them for the beauty and power they possess. And we can spend every day admiring the beauty in our peers, our elders, our children, and the vast majority of men who understand and uphold the value of women as equal partners.

When we do that, we are free. And we can get back to work.

Breathe into your body. Straighten up in your blouse. Find a trail, and watch as your feet strike the ground, passing from sun to shade and back to the sun again. A few miles in, you might begin to get tired, but even so, your spirits will lift. Rest. Eat. Stretch, and lose as much of the drama as you can along the way. It isn't serving you, but your body is.

Thieves, tucked away in the halls of power, are attempting to rob us of our autonomy, of fearlessness and joy. They are crippling our bodies by filling our hearts and minds with anxiety. If we allow that anxiety to destroy our health, we submit to their agenda. The way to rise above is to be unremittingly honest and vibrant, to revel in the experience of being alive in our bodies.

And if you get lost again, if you start beating up on yourself for being less than perfect, go to the neighborhood pool. Look for the grandmas doing water aerobics in the shallow end and the little kids splashing in their floaties. They'll show you how it's done. They'll remind you to do your best—and forget the rest.

For my part, I'll be dangling my feet in the water, thighs squished out flat, wearing a trucker hat, watching my son play. I'll try to keep my top on for now, but I'm not making any promises.

Fill in the Fact

Going forward, this body is mine, and I will honor it by taking care of it. (circle one):

True   False

Join forces with your body.
Take it back, for your own
enjoyment and your
own purposes.

Charitable and Social Justice Organizations

Below is a partial list of resources to get you connected with groups working on a variety of issues. Most of these are national, but many have search engines where you can find local resources as well. There are thousands of incredible organizations working nationwide and all over the world to make a difference. Pick one that resonates with you, and get in touch through the information below. A little time or effort can have a big impact, not only on their work, but on *your* health and sense of belonging as well.

Addiction

Angels at Risk—http://angelsatrisk.com/

Faces and Voices of Recovery—
http://facesandvoicesofrecovery.org/

Gearing Up—https://www.gearing-up.org/

Parents Helping Parents—
http://www.parentshelpingparents.info/

Relief Retreats—https://www.reliefretreats.com/

Shatterproof—https://www.shatterproof.org/

To Write Love on Her Arms—https://twloha.com/

Animal Protection

Animal Welfare Institute—https://awionline.org/

The Gentle Barn—http://www.gentlebarn.org/

Humane Farming Association—http://www.hfa.org/

Humane Society of the United States—
http://www.humanesociety.org/

Ian Somerhalder Foundation—
http://www.isfoundation.com/

The Marine Mammal Center—
http://www.marinemammalcenter.org/

Wildlife Conservation Society—https://www.wcs.org/

World Wildlife Fund—https://www.worldwildlife.org/

Arts Education

Americans for the Arts—http://www.americansforthearts.org/

Arts Education Partnership—http://www.aep-arts.org/

Geena Davis Institute on Gender in Media—
https://seejane.org/

National Endowment for the Arts—https://www.arts.gov/

Disability Rights

ADAPT—http://adapt.org/

The Arc—https://www.thearc.org/

Autism Women's Network—https://autismwomensnetwork.org/

The Autistic Self-Advocacy Network—http://autisticadvocacy.org/

National Council on Independent Living—http://www.ncil.org/

National Disability Rights Network—http://www.ndrn.org/

Special Needs Alliance—http://www.specialneedsalliance.org/

Domestic Violence

National Domestic Violence Hotline—
http://www.thehotline.org/, (800) 799-SAFE (7322)

National Resource Center on Domestic Violence—
http://www.nrcdv.org/

Partnership Against Domestic Violence—http://padv.org/

World YWCA—http://www.worldywca.org/

Eating Disorders

Body Image Movement—https://bodyimagemovement.com/

Eating Disorders Coalition—
http://www.eatingdisorderscoalition.org/

Eating Disorders Resource Center—http://edrcsv.org/

National Eating Disorders Association—
https://www.nationaleatingdisorders.org/

Project Heal—http://theprojectheal.org/

Environment

American Rivers—https://www.americanrivers.org/

Environmental Defense Fund—https://www.edf.org/

Environmental Working Group—http://www.ewg.org/

Friends of the Earth—http://www.foe.org/

Greenpeace—http://www.greenpeace.org/usa/

The Nature Conservancy—https://www.nature.org/

Ocean Conservancy—https://oceanconservancy.org/

Rainforest Alliance—http://www.rainforest-alliance.org/

Trust for Public Land—https://www.tpl.org/

Gun Safety

Americans for Responsible Solutions—
http://americansforresponsiblesolutions.org/

Brady Campaign to Prevent Gun Violence—
http://www.bradycampaign.org/

Everytown for Gun Safety—https://everytown.org/

Moms Demand Action—https://momsdemandaction.org/

Newtown Action Alliance—http://alliance.newtownaction.org/

HIV

amfAR, The Foundation for Aids Research—
http://www.amfar.org/

Elizabeth Glaser Pediatric AIDS Foundation—
http://www.pedaids.org/

Elton John AIDS Foundation—http://ejaf.org/

Keep a Child Alive—http://keepachildalive.org/

Homelessness

Homeless Shelter Directory—
http://www.homelessshelterdirectory.org/

National Alliance to End Homelessness—
http://endhomelessness.org/

National Coalition for the Homeless—
http://nationalhomeless.org/

National Health Care for the Homeless Council—
https://www.nhchc.org/

National Runaway Safeline—
https://www.1800runaway.org/, (800) RUNAWAY (786-2929)

Human Trafficking

APNEAAP Women Worldwide—http://apneaap.org/

National Human Trafficking Hotline—
https://humantraffickinghotline.org/, (888) 373-7888

Polaris Project—https://polarisproject.org/

Unlikely Heroes—https://unlikelyheroes.com/

Immigrant and Refugee Services

American Refugee Committee—http://arcrelief.org/

Council on American-Islamic Relations—
https://www.cair.com/

Families for Freedom—http://familiesforfreedom.org/

International Rescue Committee—https://www.rescue.org/

National Network for Immigrant and Refugee Rights—
http://www.nnirr.org/

Legal Services

American Civil Liberties Union (ACLU)—https://www.aclu.org/

Immigrant Legal Resource Center—https://www.ilrc.org/

Southern Poverty Law Center—https://www.splcenter.org/

LGBTQ Rights

LGBT National Help Center—http://www.glnh.org/

Human Rights Campaign (HRC)—http://www.hrc.org/

Mariposas Sin Fronteras (LGBTQ detained immigrants)—
https://mariposassinfronteras.org/

Parents, Family and Friends of Lesbians and Gays (PFLAG)—
https://www.pflag.org/

The Trevor Project (suicide prevention)—
http://www.thetrevorproject.org/

Mental Health

Center for Courage and Renewal—http://www.couragerenewal.org/

Mental Health America—http://www.mentalhealthamerica.net/

National Alliance on Mental Illness—https://www.nami.org/

National Suicide Prevention Hotline—
https://suicidepreventionlifeline.org/, (800) 273-8255

Net Neutrality

Electronic Frontier Foundation—https://www.eff.org/

Fight for the Future—https://www.fightforthefuture.org/

Free Press—https://www.freepress.net/

Global Net Neutrality Coalition—
https://www.thisisnetneutrality.org/

Public Knowledge—https://www.publicknowledge.org/

Peace

Code Pink—http://www.codepink.org/

Human Rights Watch—https://www.hrw.org/

International Crisis Group—https://www.crisisgroup.org/

Nonviolent Peaceforce—
http://www.nonviolentpeaceforce.org/

Peace Corps—https://www.peacecorps.gov/

Preemptive Love—http://www.preemptivelove.org/

Poverty

Care—http://www.care.org/

Catholic Charities—https://www.ilrc.org/

charity: water—https://www.charitywater.org/

The Hunger Project—http://www.thp.org/

International Center for Research on Women—
https://www.icrw.org/

More Than Sport—https://www.morethansport.org/

Women for Women International—
http://www.womenforwomen.org/

World Food Programme—http://www1.wfp.org/

Progressive Candidates

Emerge America—http://www.emergeamerica.org/

Emily's List—https://www.emilyslist.org/

Indivisible—https://www.indivisibleguide.com/

The New American Leaders Project—
https://www.newamericanleaders.org/

Women's Political Committee—
http://womenspoliticalcommittee.org/

Racial Justice

Black Lives Matter—http://blacklivesmatter.com/

Color of Change—https://www.colorofchange.org/

Equal Justice Initiative—https://eji.org/

NAACP (National Association for the Advancement of Colored People)—http://www.naacp.org/

National Cares Mentoring Movement—http://www.caresmentoring.org/

Showing Up for Racial Justice—http://www.showingupforracialjustice.org/

Veteran Support

Fisher House Foundation—https://www.fisherhouse.org/

Hire Heroes—https://www.hireheroesusa.org/

Homes for Our Troops—https://www.hfotusa.org/

Operation Homefront—http://www.operationhomefront.org/

Songwriting with Soldiers—http://www.songwritingwithsoldiers.org/

Voter Registration

Fair Elections Legal Network—http://fairelectionsnetwork.com/

HeadCount—https://www.headcount.org/

League of Women Voters—http://lwv.org/

Project Vote—http://www.projectvote.org/

Rock the Vote—https://www.rockthevote.com/

Voto Latino—http://votolatino.org/

Women's Health and Equality

HRSA Health Center Finder—https://findahealthcenter.hrsa.gov/

International Women's Health Coalition—https://iwhc.org/

Moms Rising—https://www.momsrising.org/

National Organization for Women—http://now.org/

National Women's Health Network—https://www.nwhn.org/

Planned Parenthood—https://www.plannedparenthood.org/

United Nations Population Fund—http://www.unfpa.org/

Women's March—https://www.womensmarch.com/

World Health Organization—http://www.who.int/en/

Further Reading

For Adults

All That Is Bitter and Sweet, by Ashley Judd with Maryanne Vollers. Ballantine Books, 2011.

The Body Keeps the Score: Brain, Mind, and Body in the Healing of Trauma, by Bessel van der Kolk, MD. Penguin Books, 2014.

Born a Crime: Stories from a South African Childhood, by Trevor Noah. Spiegel & Grau, 2016.

Broad Strokes: 15 Women Who Made Art and History (in That Order), by Bridget Quinn and Lisa Congdon (Illustrator). Chronicle, 2017.

Dear Madam President: An Open Letter to the Women Who Will Run the World, by Jennifer Palmeri. Grand Central, 2018.

Equilibrium, by Tiana Clark. Bull City Press, 2016.

Every Body Yoga: Let Go of Fear, Get on the Mat, Love Your Body, by Jessamyn Stanley. Workman Publishing, 2017.

Every Day Is a Good Day: Reflections by Contemporary Indigenous Women, by Wilma Mankiller, foreword by Gloria Steinem. Fulcrum Publishing, 2011.

The Gift of Anger: And Other Lessons from My Grandfather Mahatma Gandhi, by Arun Gandhi. Simon & Schuster, 2017.

The Laura Lea Balanced Cookbook: 120+ Everyday Recipes for the Healthy Home Cook, by Laura Lea Goldberg. Spring House Press, 2017.

Make Trouble: Standing Up, Seaking Out, and Finding the Courage to Lead—My Life Story, by Cecile Richards with Lauren Peterson. Simon & Schuster, 2018.

My Life on the Road, by Gloria Steinem. Random House, 2015.

Traveling Mercies: Some Thoughts on Faith, by Anne Lamott. Anchor, 2000.

Truth and Beauty: A Friendship, by Ann Patchett. Harper Perennial, 2005.

When Breath Becomes Air, by Paul Kalanithi. Random House, 2016.

When Things Fall Apart: Heart Advice for Difficult Times, by Pema Chödrön. Shambhala, 1997.

Yes, Please, by Amy Poehler. Dey Street Books, 2015.

For Kids

A Is for Activist, by Innosanto Nagara. Triangle Square, 2013.

The Big Book of Girl Power, by Julie Merberg. Downtown Books, 2016.

Harvesting Hope: The Story of Cesar Chavez, by Kathleen Krull. Illustrated by Yuyi Morales. HMH Books for Young Readers, 2003.

Heroes for My Daughter, by Brad Meltzer. HarperCollins, 2016.

Heroes for My Son, by Brad Meltzer. HarperCollins, 2016.

Let It Shine: Stories of Black Women Freedom Fighters, by Andrea Davis Pinkney. Illustrated by Stephen Alcorn. HMH Books for Young Readers, 2013.

Rad Women Worldwide: Artists and Athletes, Pirates and Punks, and Other Revolutionaries Who Shaped History, by Kate Schatz. Illustrated by Miriam Klein Stahl. Ten Speed Press, 2016.

She Persisted: 13 American Women Who Changed the World, by Chelsea Clinton. Illustrated by Alexandra Boiger. Philomel Books, 2017.

Strange Fruit: Billie Holiday and the Power of a Protest Song, by Gary Golio. Illustrated by Charlotte Riley-Webb. Millbrook Press, 2017.

Strong Is the New Pretty: A Celebration of Girls Being Themselves, by Kate T. Parker. Workman Publishing Company, 2017.

Women in Science: 50 Fearless Pioneers Who Changed the World, by Rachel Ignotofsky. Ten Speed Press, 2016.

Your Body Is Awesome: Body Respect for Children, by Sigrun Danielsdottier and Bjork Bjarkadottir (illustrator). Singing Dragon, 2014.

Notes

Chapter 1: Strange Beauty

1. Cohen, Leonard. 1971. "Beneath My Hands." *Selected Poems, 1956–1968*. Bantam Books.

2. McClellan, Seth, and Hetzel, Mark. 2016. *Little Wound's Warriors*. Thorne Creek Productions.

3. QuitAlcohol.com. 2016. "Addiction Treatment Policy Under President Trump." QuitAlcohol.com, https://www.quitalcohol.com/treatment/addiction-treatment-policy-president-trump.html.

Chapter 3: No Such Thing as Fearlessness

1. Tunick, Spencer. 2016. http://spencertunickcleveland.com/.

2. Center for American Women and Politics staff. 2017. "Women in Elective Office 2017." Center for American Women and Politics, Eagleton Institute of Politics, Rutgers University, http://www.cawp.rutgers.edu/women-elective-office-2017.

3. Certified Financial Planner Board of Standards. 2017. "Making More Room for Women in the Financial Planning Profession." Certified Financial Planner Board of Standards, http://www.cfp.net/docs/about-cfp-board/cfp-board_win_web.pdf?sfvrsn=2.

4. Roose, Kevin. 2015. "Survey Says: 92 Percent of Software Developers Are Men." *Splinter*, https://splinternews.com/survey-says-92-percent-of-software-developers-are-men-1793846921.

5. Warner, Judith. 2014. "Fact Sheet: The Women's Leadership Gap." Center for American Progress, https://www.americanprogress.org/issues/women/reports/2014/03/07/85457/fact-sheet-the-womens-leadership-gap.

6. Kilday, Gregg. 2017. "Study: Female Filmmakers Lost Ground in 2016." *The Hollywood Reporter*, https://www.hollywoodreporter.com/news

/women-filmmakers-2016-statistics-show-female-directors-declined
-number-963729.

7. McGregor, Jena. 2016. "This Staggering Chart Shows How Few Women Hold Executive Positions." *The Washington Post*, https://www.washingtonpost.com/news/on-leadership/wp/2016/03/30/this-staggering-chart-shows-how-few-minority-women-hold-executive-positions/?utm_term=.c628113302f5.

8. Warner, Judith. 2014. "Fact Sheet: The Women's Leadership Gap." Center for American Progress, https://www.americanprogress.org/issues/women/reports/2014/03/07/85457/fact-sheet-the-womens-leadership-gap.

9. Wikipedia. 2017. "She-Ra." *Wikipedia*, https://en.wikipedia.org/wiki/She-Ra.

Chapter 4: Bodies Don't Lie

1. Relief Retreats. 2017. https://www.reliefretreats.com.

2. Tippett, Krista. 2014. Interview with Bessel Van Der Kolk. "Restoring the Body: Yoga, EMDR, and Treating Trauma." *On Being*, NPR, https://onbeing.org/programs/bessel-van-der-kolk-restoring-the-body-yoga-emdr-and-treating-trauma.

3. Jaye, Sally. 2017. *Sally Jaye*, http://www.sallyjaye.com.

Chapter 5: Exercise

1. Belluz, Julia, and Zarracina, Javier. 2017. "Why You Shouldn't Exercise to Lose Weight, Explained with 60+ Studies." *Vox*, http://www.vox.com/2016/4/28/11518804/weight-loss-exercise-myth-burn-calories.

2. Southern Alliance for People and Animal Welfare. 2017. http://www.safpaw.org.

3. More Than Sport. 2017. https://www.morethansport.org.

4. Dove. 2016. "New Dove Research Finds Beauty Pressures Up, and Women and Girls Calling for Change." *Cision PR Newswire*, http://www.prnewswire.com/news-releases/new-dove-research-finds-beauty-pressures-up-and-women-and-girls-calling-for-change-583743391.html.

5. Tennessee Association of Vintage Base Ball. 2016. Tennessee Association of Vintage Base Ball, http://tennesseevintagebaseball.com/about-us.

Chapter 6: Food as Medicine

1. Bennett, Connie, and Sinatra, Stephen T. 2006. *Sugar Shock!: How Sweets and Simple Carbs Can Derail Your Life—And How You Can Get Back on Track*. Berkley.

2. Cohen, Rich. 2013, August. "Sugar Love: A Not So Sweet Tale." *National Geographic*.

3. Goldberg, Laura Lea. 2017. "Minty Fudge Brownie Bites & 7 Quick Snack Ideas." Laura Lea Balanced, http://llbalanced.com/recipes/minty -fudge-brownie-bites-7-quick-snack-ideas.

4. Freidman, Ron. 2014. "What You Eat Affects Your Productivity." *Harvard Business Review*, https://hbr.org/2014/10/what-you -eat-affects-your-productivity.

Chapter 7: Alternative Therapies

1. Stahl, Michael. 2017. "Blog." Peregrine Center, http://www.peregrine center.com.

2. WebMD. 2017. "Overview of Biofeedback." WebMD, http://www .webmd.com/a-to-z-guides/biofeedback-therapy-uses-benefits#1.

3. WebMD. 2017. "EMDR: Eye Movement Desensitization and Reprocessing." WebMD, http://www.webmd.com/mental-health/emdr -what-is-it#1.

4. Einstein, Albert. 1931. *Living Philosophies*. Simon and Schuster.

5. Float Nashville. 2017. Float Nashville, https://www.floatnashville.com.

6. Zhang, Xiaorui. 2002. "Acupuncture: Review and Analysis of Reports on Controlled Clinical Trials." World Health Organization, http://www .iama.edu/OtherArticles/acupuncture_WHO_full_report.pdf.

7. Einstein, Albert. 1948. *Atomic Physics*. Film. J. Arthur Rank Organization, Ltd., http://history.aip.org/history/exhibits/einstein/voice1.htm.

8. Fishman, Jon. 2017. "The History of Acupuncture." Acupuncture .com, http://www.acupuncture.com/education/theory/historyacu.htm.

9. Chiropractic care can be very useful for some people in some situations, but it simply wasn't working for my neck in this particular situation.

10. Reiki.org. 2017. "What Is Reiki?" The International Center for Reiki Training, http://www.reiki.org/faq/whatisreiki.html.

11. Jones, Bill. 1975. "Spatial Perception in the Blind." *British Journal of Psychology*, Wiley Online Library, http://onlinelibrary.wiley.com /doi/10.1111/j.2044-8295.1975.tb01481.x/abstract;jsessionid=7EBD3ED CE78F3C90FDB824FABEB02822.f04t03.

12. Zeidan, Fadel. 2016. "A Different Approach to Pain Management: Mindfulness Meditation." TEDxEmory, TEDx Talks, https://www.youtube .com/watch?v=OLQJJDrbj6Q.

Chapter 9: Motherhood

1. Pan American Development Foundation. 2017. "Preparing Girls and Women for Prosperity." Pan American Development Foundation, https://static1.squarespace.com/static/54073cece4b0bf6cd12bf4c9/t /5419c4b2e4b097579b5de0cc/1410974898317/Empowering+Girls +and+Women+for+Prosperity+%28pages%29.pdf.

2. Girls to the Moon. 2017. Girls to the Moon, https://girlstothemoon .com.

3. Moms Demand Action. 2017. Moms Demand Action for Gun Sense in America, https://momsdemandaction.org/about.

Chapter 10: Social Media

1. Full disclosure: Kate is my cousin, and I may or may not have peed in my pants more than once in her bedroom from laughing too hard.

2. Hays, Kate. 2017. http://www.northmainstrategy.com/.

3. Mayo Clinic Staff. 2016. "Miscarriage." Mayo Clinic, https://www .mayoclinic.org/diseases-conditions/pregnancy-loss-miscarriage/home /ovc-20213664.

4. Lamott, Anne. 2000. *Traveling Mercies: Some Thoughts on Faith.* Anchor.

5. Natividad, Angela. 2017. "How Dove Is 'Hacking' Photography to Change the Way Advertising Depicts Women." *Adweek*, https://www.adweek .com/creativity/how-dove-is-hacking-photography-to-change-the-way -advertising-depicts-women.

6. Café Rooster Records. https://www.caferoosterrecords.com/.

7. Stacie Huckeba Photography. https://www.staciehuckeba.com./

8. Isbell, Jason. 2017. "Hope the High Road." The Nashville Sound. http://www.jasonisbell.com/.

Chapter 11: Rest

1. Dead Horses. 2016. "Golden Sky." *Cartoon Moon*, http://www.dead horses.net/.

Chapter 13: Fragility as Practice

1. King, Martin Luther, Jr. 1959. "Farewell Statement for All India Radio." Transcript of audio recording. The Martin Luther King Jr. Papers Project, Stanford University, http://kingencyclopedia.stanford.edu/primarydocuments /Vol5/9Mar1959_FarewellStatementforAllIndiaRadio.pdf.

Chapter 14: Keep It Interesting

1. Bliss, Jessica. 2017. "The Desegregation of Nashville Schools—And the Bombing That Followed 60 Years Ago." *The Tennessean*, http://www .tennessean.com/story/news/education/2017/09/08/desegregation -nashville-schools-and-bombing-followed-60-years-ago/637665001/.

Acknowledgments

To all of my clients and friends who fell apart on the day we woke up to find that misogyny and discrimination had been sanctioned to a degree we never imagined possible, thank you for staying honest with yourselves and with me. You showed me in those first few months what defeat turned inward looks like—and then I watched you step up and stand tall, one by one. You keep me sane and keep me moving every day. Thank you.

To Ken, Sky, and Ringo, you guys need to revive the vaudeville circuit and take the show on the road. Thank you for letting me be quiet while you tumble through the world. You never let a day go by without making me laugh, even if it involves sliding small objects under my office door when I've locked you out. I love you madly.

Mom and Dad, you are an inspiration. You have taught me the arts of forward motion and quiet reflection, and I am forever grateful for both.

To the women who have shaped me: Jana, Tracy, JJ, Sally, Katrina, Martha, Jessica, Linnet, Lindsay, Traci, Marcia, Emily R., Emily H., Jennifer, Kate, Sumeeta, Debbie, Marna, Lisa, Julia, Katy, and Annie, you are home base. Thank you for always saying the right thing at the right time, even if that thing is hard to hear. I would be a lost soul and a bumbling mother if it weren't for every one of you. I hope you can see the beauty and power in yourselves that I see plain as day.

Allison Cohen, I have no idea what I did to deserve you. I also don't totally believe that you're not at least partially bionic. You are a force. Thank you for four years of unwavering support and for coaching me to step away when I'm climbing the walls. This book and the one before it would have been impossible without you.

Stephanie Knapp, thank you for giving me free rein to rant from the gut and for believing that physical well-being is both powerful and political. I'm so thankful there are women like you curating the words we read on the page and the books that sit on our bookshelves.

Seal Press, you publish books that give voice to a diverse, irreverent, irrepressible group of women. Thank you for being a megaphone for feminism and for including me in the chorus. I couldn't have asked for a better match.

There were so many people who spent hours telling me about their personal and professional struggles and triumphs. I wish I could have included every one of their stories here because every one helped shape this book. Thank you for taking the time to talk with me.

Last, thanks to the women and allies leading the charge in entertainment, politics, business, and education to shape our media diets, the laws that govern us, and the opportunities available to women and girls. You are reinforcing our lives from all sides, and we have your backs. Keep calm and carry on!

About the Author

Personal trainer and "diet abolitionist," Sarah Hays Coomer, is the author of *Lightness of Body and Mind: A Radical Approach to Weight and Wellness*. She is a Certified Personal Trainer with the National Strength and Conditioning Association and a Certified Nutrition and Wellness Consultant and Pre/Postnatal Fitness Specialist with American Fitness Professionals & Associates. Her work has been featured in *Shape*, *MSN*, *The Wall Street Journal*, *New York Daily News*, *The Tennessean*, *Bustle*, and *LifeHack*, among others. She kind of likes to exercise, kind of not. Sarah lives and trains in Nashville with her husband, son, and sweet pit bull, Ringo.

• • •

The author will donate 10 percent of the royalties after payment of her agency fee and Hachette's recoupment of advances received from Hachette for sale of this book in the United States during the first year from publication as follows: 50 percent to Planned Parenthood Action Fund, and 50 percent, to the World Food Programme.